SPARTANAT BLACK BOOK 4

SPARTANAT

spartanat.com

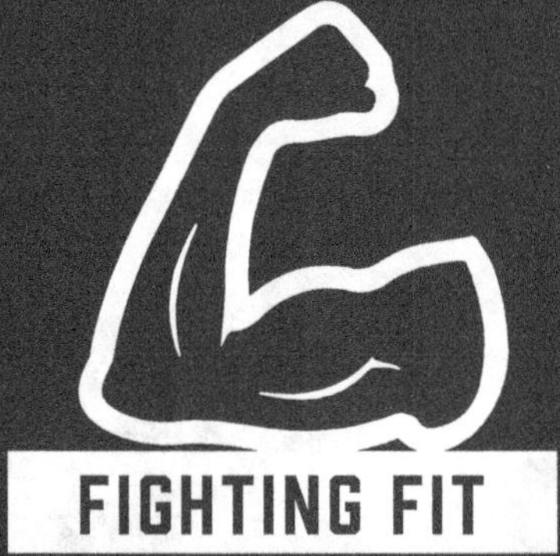

Doktor-Herrmann-Gasse 4
9020 Klagenfurt am Wörthersee, Austria

ISBN 978-3-903526-08-2

FIGHTING FIT

// SPECIAL FORCES FITNESS

// GET READY FOR GERMAN NAVY SEALS / KAMPFSCHWIMMER

// EFFECTIVE TRAINING TO MEET SOF ENTRY REQUIREMENTS

TORSTEN SCHREIBER

TABLE OF CONTENTS

INTRODUCTION

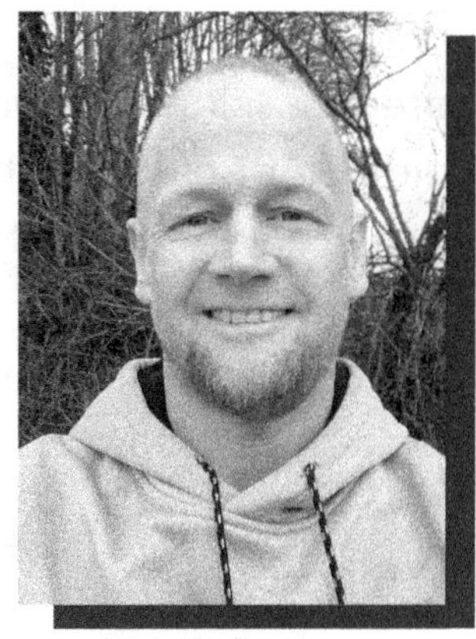

The training plans views, and statements in this book are based on my own personal experience. My name is Torsten Schreiber. I have been a "Kampfschwimmer" – a German Navy SEAL in Eckernförde – since 2003 and, together with Andreas Aumann, wrote the book *Military Fitness: Training Like A Kampfschwimmer.*

I have been doing triathlons since 1995 and have involved myself in all types of sports for even longer (climbing, weights, SwimRun ÖTILLÖ, adventure races, ball games, and many more). This has enabled me to acquire extensive knowledge, which, on occasion, deviates from current doctrine. Unfortunately, the individuality factor in sports is often ignored.

Many people dream of being a member of an elite team. Many have what it takes, but only a few make it. Why is that? During my time as an instructor in the training inspectorate of the Eckernförde "Kampfschwimmerkompanie", I was privileged to meet and work with numerous of candidates.

Most fail on the first day or during the first week. This is partly due to substandard or unsound physical preparation.

Of course, many are also forced to give up due to other problems, regardless of their physical fitness. Mental stamina plays the second-biggest role in preparation. Quite often, a misconception of the dream assignment or private issues also lead to candidates throwing in the towel. These are all aspects that are very difficult for individuals to influence.

However, the physical fitness required to meet the entry requirements and to be well-prepared later in the training program is not an insurmountable concern. And that is exactly what we want to tackle in this book.

There are some training plans that are exclusively designed to meet entrance requirements. Passing the entrance test only means that you can start the training program. Most units, however, demand much more than what has to be achieved in the tests.

That is why I recommend that you make sure that your fitness level is always much higher than that required to (barely) pass the tests. However, I do not want to raise false hopes, which is why I say that a book, a booklet, or an online training plan will never be enough to achieve maximum performance. Many publishers of training plans unfortunately make this promise. However, with all-inclusive training plans you have to factor in personal aspects, which only a custom-made training plan by a trainer can cover.

This booklet is an all-in-one package and should be seen as a kind of guideline. It is up to you to incorporate your abilities and weaknesses into your weekly planning, because these are the factors that I cannot take into account here. If the units required in the book are below the standard of your abilities, then train what you are used to and with a training load you can cope with without overexertion. Use the following advice and plans as a basis, but remain flexible in your training plans. If you have the chance, always ask a trainer or experienced athlete to observe your training in order to get input for improvement. Please read the entire booklet before you start with the training plans, as the individual chapters contain important information on various units. This can spare you a lot of questions.

Good luck!

IMPORTANT INSTRUCTIONS:

- ***We offer no liability for injuries; you complete the training plan at your own risk.***
- ***Consult a physician before starting such an extensive plan and get a proper medical check-up.***
- ***Training when you are ill can lead to serious health issues.***
- ***It is better to skip a few sessions and only start again when you are feeling better.***
- ***If you have any questions, you can always contact me via Instagram: www.instagram.com/todde_439***

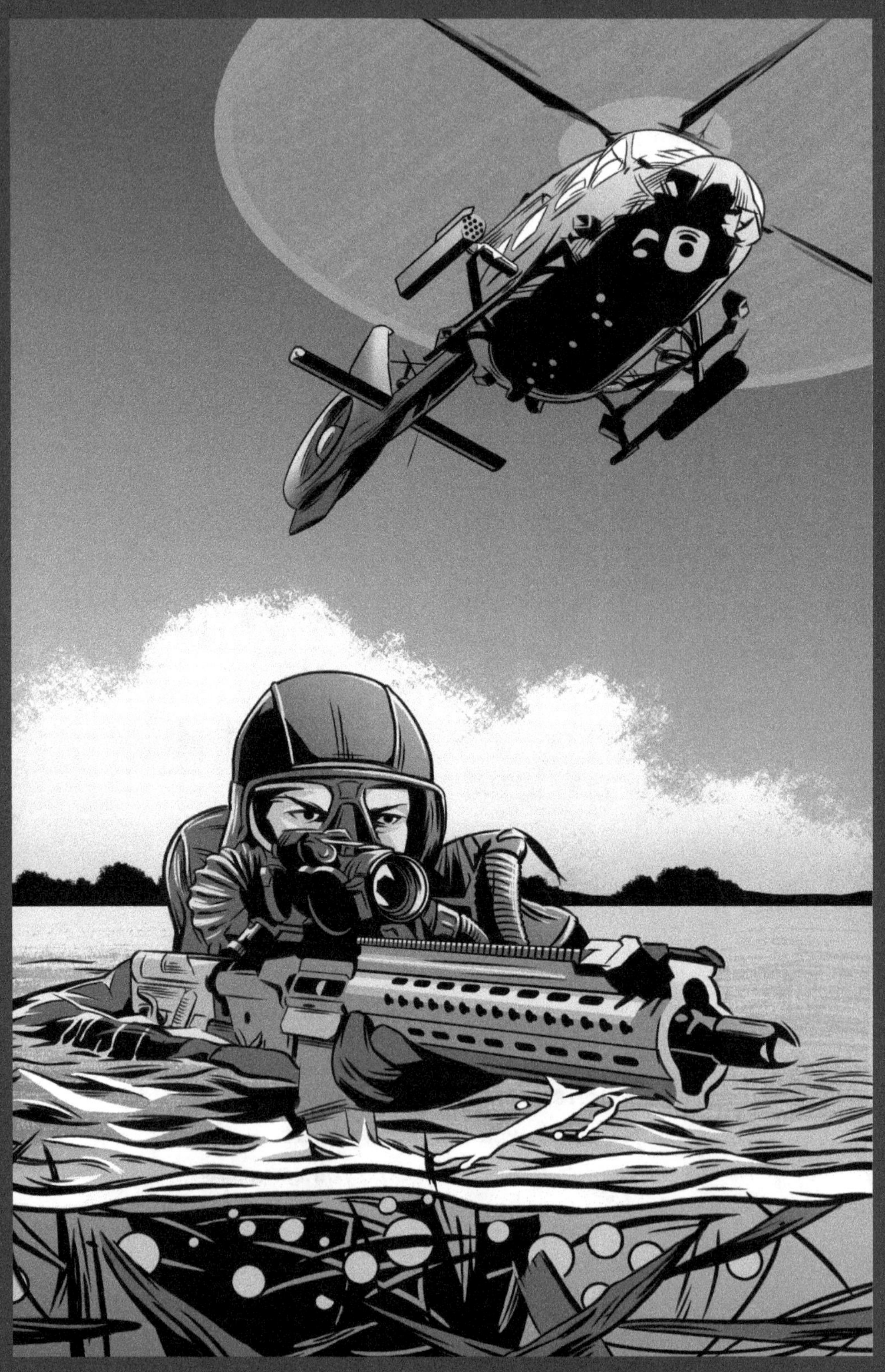

SPECIAL OPERATIONS FORCES

1

WHAT ARE SPECIAL FORCES?

"Who Dares Wins" is the motto of the British Special Air Service, which was formed during the Second World War and remains one of the world's finest special operations forces. The SAS was the model for all Special Operations Forces (SOF) in the western world, and later also for the American Special Forces (SF), which were established during the Vietnam War.

"Who Dares Wins" is the perfect motto for soldiers who are relied upon to accomplish exceptionally important and extremely dangerous missions. SOF basically employ "normal" soldiers; the demands on them, however, are incomparably higher and more specialized. The special forces soldier, the so-called operator, is the top athlete among soldiers, so to speak, which can be understood quite literally. Due to the high physical demands, these soldiers are also referred to as **tactical athletes**. Special forces are therefore operationally a strategic, high-value instrument in the hands of military and political leaders. Wherever these units are deployed, the aim is to achieve a lot and attract little attention. Operations are often secret and sometimes spectacular. Sometimes a few individuals are expected to achieve what many cannot. Special forces can also be force multipliers, i.e., forces that develop and build up force in order to intervene. The range of tasks perfectly illustrates how these soldiers are employed:

Direct Action ▶ *brings force to the enemy, direct combat operation.*
Special Reconnaissance ▶ *gathers information, conducts special reconnaissance for the operational level.*
Military Assistance ▶ *refers to training operations abroad.*
Close Protection ▶ *is personal protection.*
Hostage Rescue and Recovery ▶ *means freeing hostages and taking them to safety.*
Counterterrorism ▶ *means fighting terrorism.*
Unconventional Warfare ▶ *means guerrilla warfare.*
Covert Operations ▶ *are operations that take place inconspicuously and secretly.*

Guerrilla warfare and terrorism can be regarded as forms of unconventional warfare. Special military and police units are often the forces confronting these threats.

KOMMANDO SPEZIALKRÄFTE MARINE [KSM] 1/1

GERMAN NAVAL SPECIAL FORCES COMMAND

Germany's oldest SOF. Its combat swimmers must fulfill tasks both in water and on land, just like the German frogmen in the Second World War. What was new was their deployment from the air as parachutists. This triphibian concept, adopted from the French, became the basis for the German Navy's combat swimmers.

Since 1972, a personnel exchange program has been in place between the combat swimmers and their American counterpart, the United States Navy SEALs, in order to further develop equipment, operational procedures, and training.

On April 1, 1964, the "Kampfschwimmer" were merged into an independent company that was subordinated to the amphibious group of the German Navy. The "Kampfschwimmer" have been stationed at Eckernförde naval base since 1974. In October 1991, they were subordinated to the Mine Warfare Flotilla and integrated into the Armed Swimmer Group. In consequence of a reorganization of the Navy that began in 2001, the "Kampfschwimmer Company" was subordinated to the Specialized Task Forces of the Navy (SEK M) in July 2003. In April 2014, the "Kampfschwimmer" formed the **Naval Special Forces Command (KSM)**.

TASKS OF THE GERMAN NAVY SEALS

▸ ***Direct Action (DA)***

Offensive, targeted operations, restricted in terms of space and time, to capture/rescue people, take possession of, destroy, or damage material/facilities, while avoiding collateral damage.

DA is directed against high-value targets. For example, to capture individuals, such as war criminals or bomb makers, who threaten German soldiers with their explosive devices or other means. They are also directed against objects or facilities. On land, these are buildings, at sea, these are ships or oil rigs which are seized using a procedure called Visit Board Search and Seizure (VBSS). VBSS is one of the procedures at which combat swimmers are particularly adept. This is because they can attack above and below water or from the air.

▸ ***Special Reconnaissance (SR)***

Operations to obtain specific, clearly defined, and time-critical information of strategic and operational importance. Examples of maritime special reconnaissance:

– Reconnaissance of harbor facilities. Combat swimmers infiltrate harbors underwater and remain undetected by the enemy.

- Reconnaissance of littoral areas, where they gather information about the nature of the beaches and the coastline.
- Reconnaissance in the hinterland, in which they approach the coast diving or swimming, explore the hinterland to discover possible dangers, and alert their own forces.

▸ ***Military Assistance (MA)***

Military operations providing direct/indirect support, to improve domestic/national security and the stability of states.

This means training the military or police units of friendly states, which can take place domestically or internationally.

More information on the KSM:
www.bundeswehr.de/de/organisation/marine/organisation/einsatzflottille-1/kommando-spezialkraefte-marine

KOMMANDO SPEZIALKRÄFTE [KSK]

GERMAN SPECIAL FORCES COMMAND

1/2

The KSK is a unit of the German Army which carries out special operations in the context of national and alliance defense as well as crisis prevention and crisis management.

Its mission includes reconnaissance and surveillance of important military targets in crisis and conflict areas, combined with the gathering of important information about enemy forces. It may also be necessary to rescue German citizens from war and civil war zones, or to free them in a hostage situation, or to free German soldiers who have been taken prisoner or hostage and return them to their unit.

More information on the KSK:
www.bundeswehr.de/de/aktuelles/schwerpunkte/spezialkraefte-bundeswehr/kommando-spezialkraefte

1/3

SPEZIALEINSATZ-KOMMANDO [SEK]

SPECIAL TASK FORCES OF GERMAN POLICE

SEKs, like the GSG 9 of the German Federal Police, were established after the terrorist attack during the 1972 Olympics in Munich.

As a result of these events, in 1974, the Standing Conference of Interior Ministers and Senators adopted the Concept for the Establishment and Employment of Special Units of the Federal States and the Federal Government to Combat Terrorists. This decision can be viewed as the birth of the special police units in Germany.

Their tasks are

- Counter-Terrorism
- Hostage rescue and seizure
- Deployment in particularly dangerous situations
- Execution of arrest warrants
- Prevention of suicide attempts
- Escorting prisoner transports
- Raids on organised crime
- Personal and witness protection measures

GRENZSCHUTZGRUPPE 9 DER BUNDESPOLIZEI [GSG 9]

BORDER GUARD GROUP 9 OF THE FEDERAL POLICE [GSG 9]

Unlike in most other countries, GSG 9 was not formed from existing military special forces, which has historical reasons. GSG 9 was created after the bloody hostage crisis during the 1972 Olympics in Munich.

Ulrich Wegener, a lieutenant colonel in the Federal Border Guard, who had previously worked as a liaison officer for the Federal Border Guard at the Federal Ministry of the Interior, was tasked by Secretary of the Interior Hans-Dietrich Genscher with setting up a powerful anti-terrorist unit. In April 1973, Wegener announced the operational readiness of two GSG 9 units.

The name GSG 9 can be explained by the structure of the Federal Border Guard at the time, which consisted of four Border Guard Commands with a total of eight Border Guard Groups (GSG 1 to 7 and Sea) when this unit was founded. As GSG 9 was not integrated into any of the existing structures, it was given the designation Border Guard Group 9.

1/4

It retained this designation and the status of a border guard group during the reorganisations of the Federal Border Guard.

The tasks of GSG 9:

- Counter-Terrorism
- Hostage rescue
- EOD
- Combating serious crime

More information on the GSG 9:
www.bundespolizei.de/Web/DE/05Die-Bundespolizei/04Einsatzkraefte/GSG9-neu/gsg9_node.html

JAGDKOMMANDO –
AUSTRIAN ARMED FORCES COMMANDOS

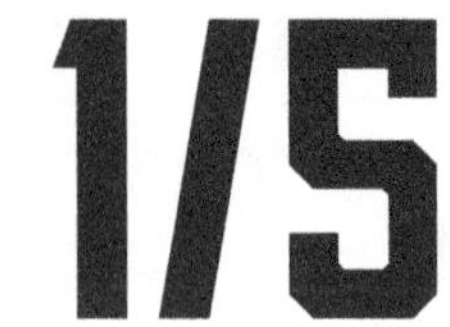

In 1963, the order was given to organize the first Commando basic course, and the "Jagdkommando" was set up as a company. At that time, the aim of the newly launched training program was to continue small-scale combat in enemy-occupied territory with regular forces, the so-called commandos. In 1965, parachute training was integrated into the third basic commando course for the first time.

In 1969, training was expanded to include combat swimmer training and, in the mid-1970s, long-range reconnaissance and special operations of all kinds.

Since 1976, the Commandos have been based in Wiener Neustadt. Today, the "Jagdkommando" is the initial response force and anti-terrorism unit of the Austrian Armed Forces ("Bundesheer").

The tasks of the Commandos:

- Special reconnaissance
- Commando raids
- Military support
- Military evacuation operations

More information on the Jagdkommando:
www.bundesheer.at/unser-heer/organisation/verbaende/jagdkommando

1/6

KOMMANDO SPEZIALKRÄFTE – SWISS SPECIAL FORCES COMMAND (SFC)

The "Kommando Spezialkräfte" (KSK) of Switzerland comprises the Grenadier Battalions, the KSK HQ Battalion, the Para Reconnaissance Company 17, the Armed Forces Reconnaissance Detachment 10 (AAD 10), the Military Police Special Detachment (MP Spez Det) and the Special Forces Training Centre (AZ SK). The KSK comprises professional and militia components. The KSK ensures the maintenance, training and further development of precision marksmanship, military parachuting, survival techniques and survival in the field, heliborne techniques, explosive entry techniques, amphibious infiltration techniques, personal protection, and intervention. The Special Forces Training Center (AZ SK) is both the training center for the special forces and the center of excellence for the entire armed forces. The KSK's range of services includes:

- Protection and interventions in support of the civilian authorities in Switzerland
- Special reconnaissance and direct actions in support of the civilian authorities or in support of the Joint Operations Command (in the event of a heightened threat situation in Switzerland)

More information on the KSK CH:
www.armee.ch/ksk

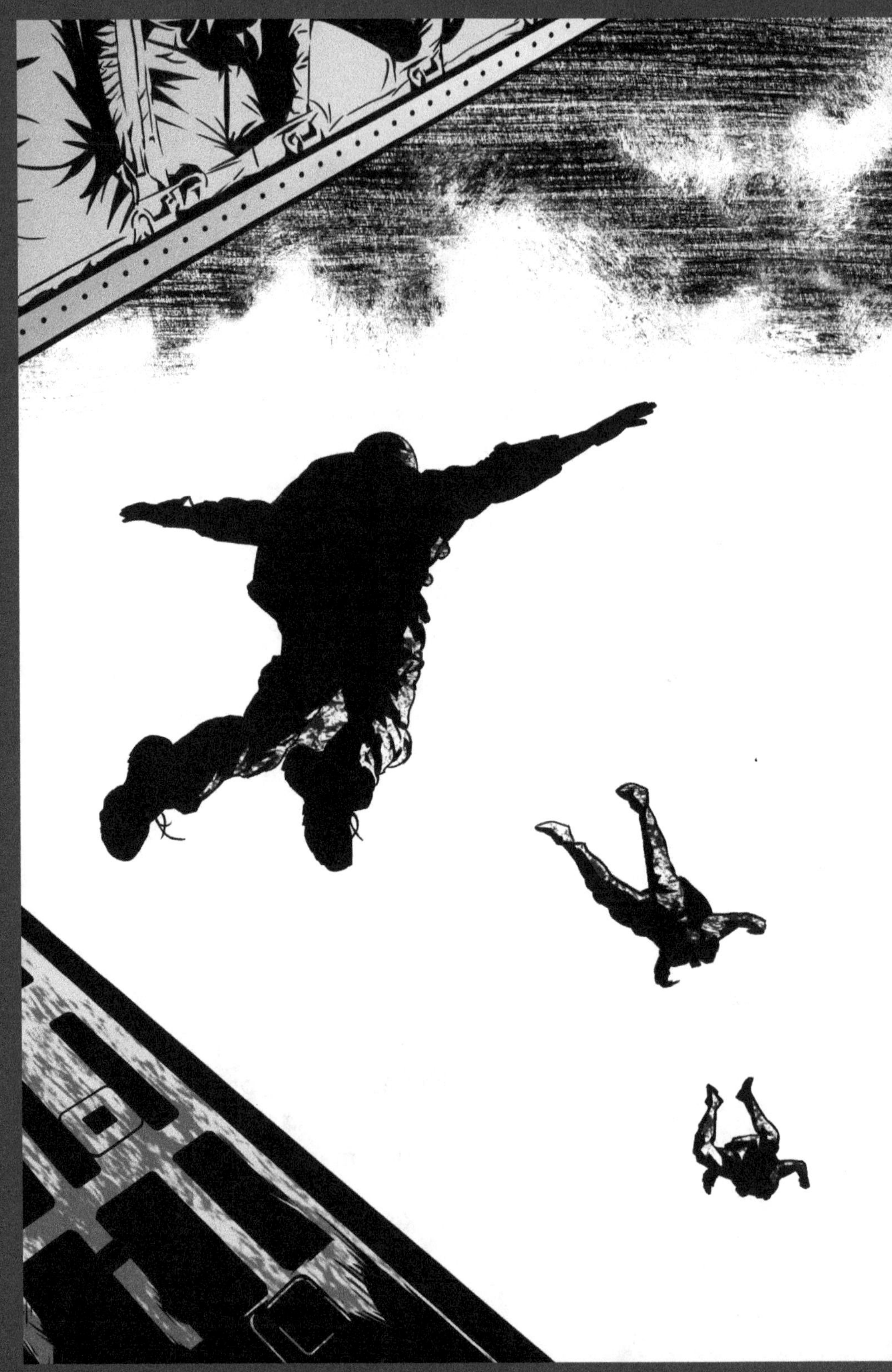

TRAINING BASICS

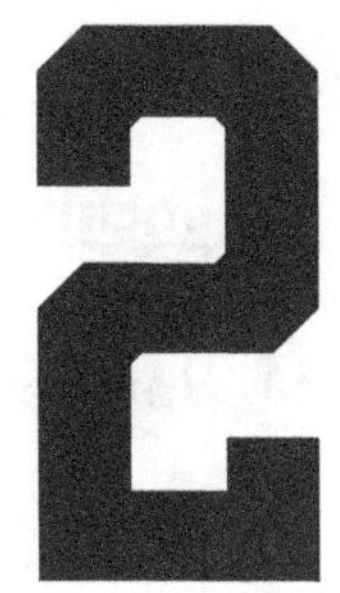

LEARN TO SUFFER PAIN WITHOUT COMPLAINING

"Lerne Leiden ohne zu klagen." This is the motto of the combat "Kampfschwimmer" program. The motto says it all. The Navy is not alone in demanding absolute resilience.

It is the principle of all special operations forces. Therefore, always remember one fact: SOFs are not looking for a top athlete; they want to recruit young, capable individuals able to push themselves beyond their limits and not give up when it hurts. If they also happen to be excellent athletes, so much the better for the units.

That does not mean you should not prepare. If you can run better, swim faster, and carry heavier weights than the rest of the training course, you will have a much easier time or can even gather valuable points that will look good in your assessments, training, and activity reports.

Practical examples

- While others are running at their limit, a fast runner can rest and save "grit" for the next exercise.
- It is easy for good swimmers with a good sense of the water to remain on the surface while holding a 10-pound ring in their hands. Poor swimmers can experience massive problems. They get out of breath and their muscles acidify, making all further exercises increasingly difficult.
- Well-trained athletes will find it relatively easy to carry fully packed rucksacks for hours as their well-developed muscles can cope with the weight. A physically weaker course participant, however, will lose a lot of strength and will require considerably more recovery time afterwards, which is rare during training.

IS THERE A BEST SPORT OR A BEST PREREQUISITE FOR PASSING THESE TESTS?

To prepare yourself optimally for training, you need to consider a few points. Many athletes like to train their strengths and tend to neglect their weaknesses. Do not make this mistake. Being good at everything is better than being the best in one discipline and the weakest link in another.

Physical appearance hardly plays a role here. I have trained a wide variety of students. From the wiry runner to the muscular athlete to the spongy all-rounder. I realized that looks mean little. Because anyone can successfully complete this training if they are willing and their physical fitness is good.

Examples of different types of exercise:

The following observations only deal with physical abilities. I will ignore the mental aspect for now.

- In my experience, a well-trained **gym athlete** with mountains of muscle has the least chance to survive a long and enduring training program. This is because the sports units focus almost exclusively on strength-endurance. This is not advantageous to musclemen, as their muscles fatigue very quickly because they have been trained primarily for speed-strength. Of course, exceptions prove the rule here, too.

- **Wiry runners** who run five kilometers in under 18 minutes will face hardly any problems in most exercises. Heavy rucksacks, boots, and other weights will, however, prove their undoing, because their low weight, coupled with little muscle mass, cannot deal with such loads. What is more, the weight loss, which inevitably occurs when training lasts several weeks or months, has a massive impact on this type of athlete.

- **Triathletes** are versatile athletes, quite good at running and swimming tests. Cycling also helps them in the ergometer tests. These endurance athletes are usually weak in strength exercises, as triathletes only do strength-endurance exercises. However, their competition experience has taught them to push themselves, which is an important factor.

- **All-round athletes** represent a very good combination. These are often athletes who have never been able to decide on one specific sport and thus try to have a finger in all sports pies, or who always do other sports in addition to their main sport. Because they enjoy variety, love all aspects of sports, and are adept at everything, they may never be the best at one sport, but they are good at all of them. For example, they have been active in the gym for several years, but also enjoy jogging. If they enjoyed swimming when younger, they will find it much easier to start swimming training than non-swimmers. They go climbing for a change or do martial arts—all good sports which create the best preconditions.

WHAT DO THESE FINDINGS MEAN FOR US?

It is possible that people spend years unconsciously preparing for such training. As a result, they have created very good basic conditions because they do not really have to think about pure sport. Other athletes, however, hardly benefit from their years of training. Take, for example, very good badminton players. Their stamina, strength, and speed are ideally suited to their sport, but will only help them to a limited extent in SOF training.

So, first and foremost, pay attention to the demands that will be placed on you. Just because you are fit does not mean that you can pass every test or undergo extreme training. Depending on your performance, you should choose an appropriate time frame before applying for an SOF, because individuals who have failed once often do not try again. This is a great pity, because some applicants simply lack the effective training they would need to progress.

HOW LONG WILL IT TAKE ME TO PREPARE FOR TRAINING?

This question is often made light of. For several years now, I have been working with young people who have set themselves the goal of becoming a member of the special forces or a "Kampfschwimmer". I draft training plans and complete training sessions with them to look at running techniques or explain important health aspects of training. They include a wide variety of characters and athletes. We have to differentiate between beginners, advanced sportspeople, and "professionals." Depending on individual performance, preparation can take anywhere between six months and a year and a half.

Beginners will have a very difficult time. These are young individuals who have hardly any sporting experience. There is always one candidate whom I would classify in this category. Unfortunately, in addition to their physical abilities, their willpower is also not up to scratch. Here, too, exceptions prove the rule. I recommend that anyone who feels that this is him complete an extended basic sports program and perhaps gain initial experience in an infantry unit, such as the paratroopers in the Bundeswehr. Experience in the military, but above all in sports, allows you to prepare yourself in a focused manner since the armed forces usually provide enough time for sport. It is a great pity when beginners fail the test, draw the wrong conclusions, and do not try again, even though they would be perfectly capable of becoming good operators with the help of a sensible training plan.

The advanced athletes are always my favorites. These athletes have already gained experience in jogging, strength training, swimming, and other interesting sports. Their bodies are used to stress, and they know something about training theory. After a short basic training program, the advanced athletes can go straight into a targeted build-up training program. Depending on individual performance, 6 to 12 months are realistic.

"Pros" are very good athletes who have also done a lot of work on the subject of special forces. They no longer need training in running, weights, or swimming. Their times are excellent. They want to go one step further and prepare for the training weeks because they are sure to meet the minimum requirements. I can run through specific training sessions with them to prepare them for the hard training, such as: **carrying tree trunks**, **apnea exercises**, **rucksack runs,** or **combined running and strength units**.

IS IT ENOUGH TO MEET THE MINIMUM REQUIREMENTS?

Let us compare the times required for combat swimmer recruits with my experiences from my time as an instructor.

▶ 5,000 METERS RUN IN UNDER 22 MINUTES

Anyone who is not able to beat this time by several minutes should work hard on their running skills. After all, running is part of everyday service and operations, at least in military units. During training, the recruits' times usually settle down at 18–20 minutes. Of course, there are also faster runners. However, 19–20 minutes is a pretty good time.

▶ 1,000 METERS SWUM IN UNDER 24 MINUTES

In my opinion, this is an almost ridiculous time. A very good swimmer is able to swim the 1,000 meters in 12–14 minutes. I have even seen 11 minutes in Eckernförde. Even good swimmers can do the distance in around 15–16 minutes. The slower ones take around 18–20 minutes.

But there are still poor swimmers who have performed well in all other areas of training and have become part of the unit in the end. Nevertheless, a good swimmer has a better chance. With a good sense of the water, they also have fewer problems in the tests and during training.

▶ 8 PULL-UPS

I do not need to say much about this. Strength training is always part of the game because of the heavy equipment and weapons. It is not necessary to strive for a bodybuilder figure, which is almost always depicted as standard in Hollywood films about SOF. But eight pull-ups are rather embarrassing.

▶ 15 X 100-POUNDS BENCH PRESS

Here, I would like to repeat what I said in my statement about pull-ups. This should be surpassed many times over.

▶ 60-SECOND STATIC APNEA

You should aim for two minutes during preparation, because the times you have to achieve during training will steadily increase in the first few weeks.

▶ 30 METERS DIVE WITH TURN

The same applies as with static apnea. The distances increase from week to week, so it is better to train for 50 meters to start your training in a relaxed manner. Please always remember to carry out all diving training sessions in pairs.

If you pass out, you will end up at the bottom of the pool. This has even happened to apnea professionals who just wanted to dive a few short distances, which, in normal circumstances, they could exceed by far. In combat swimmer training, recruits regularly pass out. So I know what I'm talking about.

▶ CONCLUSION

Minimum requirements should be seen as just that. Unfortunately, I have found that many recruits have the wrong idea and tend to regard these requirements as a good average. These recruits leave the training center on the very first day.

Prepare yourself and massively surpass or undercut minimum requirements. During training, your body and mind will develop, and your limits will inevitably shift. Even under maximum stress, your performance will continue to improve. This shows that you are nowhere near the limits of your ability. Everyone has the odd weak discipline. That is not a bad thing. It is normal. In these cases, the instructors want to see that you will still go beyond your limits and fight until you drop. With an attitude like that, times and scores are almost irrelevant.

▶ OVERTRAINING

In addition to the men I have prepared for SOF, I train a weekly sports group in running and strength-endurance. Especially here, with "normal" athletes, it is very easy to identify who trains too much, too hard, but above all, without enough regeneration. The body can cope very well with training at the limit for quite a while, even for several months.

But suddenly, the performance stagnates. The curve no longer goes up; it falls. This phenomenon is often misinterpreted. The athlete thinks that they have reached a point where they need to train more and, above all, harder. This is a big mistake and can have fatal consequences. The body suffers massively, and weeks go by before you discover why.

It takes weeks or months to recover from overtraining. So much for the SOF dream. You will not be able to apply again until the following year because, physically, you are a wreck if you are overtrained. Take a look at my training plans. Especially the regeneration phases. I work in accordance with an old, but very effective, principle, the so-called 2:1 or 3:1 rule.

I myself have been training in accordance with this principle for over 20 years, and my performance is improving even at my age as an over-40 athlete.

RUNNING WORKOUT

During my time as a triathlete, I always had to train for several sports. This is similar to what you will find in your schedule in the months prior to the entry test, or before you start training.

Because you have to do strength training and swimming as well as running, I would start with three running sessions per week. Two runs should be at a relaxed pace. I would cover 10–12 kilometers. The third training unit is the interval unit. Intervals only take up 5–10 percent of training time per week. This is why one session per week is enough for us. The best place to do this is on a sports field. This is because you also have to pass the tests here, and you always face the same conditions.

During the interval session, you warm up for 10 minutes. The main part is a unit performed at the limit, e.g., 4 × 1,000 meters with a break of approximately 2 minutes. You then cool down for 5–10 minutes. You can find other interval training options in the next section. Repeat this method for three weeks and then do a so-called RECOM week. More on this later.

▶ INTERVAL TRAINING OPTIONS FOR RUNNING

Since most applicants have to prepare for 3,000 m or 5,000 m runs, we can choose intervals from 100 m to 1,000 m. However, as training should also be fun, I will show you a few possible variations.

Basically, you warm up for about 10 minutes, then comes the **main part**, and then you cool down for about 5–10 minutes. The breaks between the intervals should be **rewarding breaks**. This, however, depends on the pulse range. As the **heart rate (HR)** is very individual, it is not possible to give a concrete number here. You can read more about this under the section Rewarding Break.

POSSIBLE MAIN PARTS:

3–6 × 1,000 m
4–7 × 800 m
5–10 × 400 m

---

100 m / 200 m / 400 m / 800 m / 400 m / 200 m / 100 m
200 m / 400 m / 800 m / 1,000 m / 800 m / 400 m / 200 m

Stair runs

Mountain sprints

You can use the hills/mountains on your running track to complete 10–30 second intervals. Having reached the top, trot again at a comfortable pace. Do not use extremely steep ascents for the hill sprints.

▶ THE RECOM WEEK: REGENERATION AND COMPENSATION

The RECOM week is the most important week in a four-week training program. You train hard for three weeks, with intervals. During the RECOM week, you slow down your body in a targeted manner. You only do a total of two to three easy training sessions on the bike or in the swimming pool. A very easy run of 30–35 minutes is also fine. You need to feel like you are not doing enough. But this week is crucial. It protects you from overtraining and ensures that your performance can continue to improve.

The RECOM week does not have to be a seven-day week. Five days of recovery are also sufficient, always depending on the individual level of performance. The plans are designed to cover several weeks and should be customized by you. The following applies: Listen to your body. Take a look at the term "overcompensation" in the following section. This describes how we can improve. As I pointed out earlier, there were a few athletes in my sports group who poked fun at this RECOM week or did not understand it. They had to pay the price after 4–6 six months: loss of performance, illness, and depression. Factors you should not have to deal with in the recruitment test. Without the RECOM week, your body would constantly be at its limit, which is not the right way to go in the long term.

▶ OVERCOMPENSATION

I have taken up this issue because most people do not realize that this scheme is outdated and has been revised. However, these revisions have gone so far that a normal athlete without extensive knowledge of training theory and the various technical terms can no longer work with it. In my opinion, the new model is only for specialized personnel and mainly helps professional trainers of competitive and high-performance athletes. The old model of overcompensation was based on the recovery phase. A new training stimulus should be set at a certain point in time. Unfortunately, muscles, tendons, ligaments, etc. regenerate at different speeds, which means that the old principle does not work since it advocated a sweeping view of regeneration. In addition, factors such as age, sex, condition—trained or untrained—were not taken into account.

Nevertheless, I use the model to teach my sports students that it is important never to neglect the periods of regeneration. Most people train too much rather than too little. You always have to listen to your body when setting a new training stimulus. I have often skipped a session because I did not feel up to it, but I have also done a second or third session in a day because it just felt right. Be smart, use your head, and listen to your body. Then you are most likely doing it right.

▶ THE REWARDING BREAK

The rewarding break describes the break between training intervals, but also between training sessions. At this point, we are only interested in the break between runs during interval training. We are aiming for a time when the recovery phase is not yet fully completed. This means that you should choose your break so that you have reached approximately 60–65 percent of your **maximum heart rate (HR)**.

Here is a sample calculation:

Your maximum heart rate is 175 beats per minute. 65 percent of this rate means your heart rate is 113 bpm. Now is the time to start the next interval.

▶ TRAINING ZONES AND PERCENTAGE DISTRIBUTION

I differentiate between four zones in running workouts. There are other systems as well by now. My experience with this system has been very good, and I have therefore stuck with it. For advanced runners, I would also include the **development zone**. However, this issue is not necessary here and is therefore not addressed.

RECOM recovery sessions (60–65 percent of max HR):
easy units for regeneration.

BE1 // BASIC ENDURANCE ZONE 1 (65–80 percent of HR): This type of training should be easy.

BE2 // BASIC ENDURANCE ZONE 2 (80–95 percent of HR): This type of training is brisk; speaking while training should be quite difficult.

CSE // COMPETITION-SPECIFIC ENDURANCE (95–100 percent): Training on the verge of or even at the personal performance limit.

In addition, these zones are divided into **extensive (ext.)** and **intensive (int.)**. BE2 extensive is thus a brisk run, during which the pace can still be increased. BE1 intensive is a relaxed run, which is close to BE2. It is therefore advisable to train with a heart rate monitor to avoid unintentionally training in a different zone.

In addition to regeneration (the RECOM phase), the following distribution is crucial to effective training: Some athletes (so-called training world champions) almost always train in the BE2 zone. Hardly any running units are done in the easy BE1 zone, although, at 60–70 percent, this should be the most common. It may be difficult to restrain yourself, but it is important. This is because the body then learns to work in different zones and can also better complete the fast units. The pyramid describes all training sessions in a certain period of time, e.g., 2 weeks. It states that:

5–10 percent of the training should be in the CSE zone,
20–35 percent should be in the BE2 zone, and
60–70 percent of the training should be in the BE1 zone.

For example, you could complete 5–6 BE1 runs, 1 or 2 BE2 runs, and 1 CSE run within 2 weeks.

▶ DETERMINING THE MAXIMUM HEART RATE [HRMAX]

If you want your training runs to be successful, you need to know your maximum heart rate. In other words, you need to know how high your heart rate is at maximum effort. This is because all training zones are individual and therefore expressed as percentages. You need to convert the percentage values and pay attention to them during your training runs.

Example: Let's assume that your HRmax is 200 bpm. If you are supposed to train in the BE1 zone on one day (i.e., at 65–80 percent of your HRmax), you need to jog at a heart rate of 130–160 bpm.

As your HRmax decreases over the course of your life, you should take a new test every 5 years to ensure that you always train in your optimal zone. Beginners change their HRmax quite quickly in the initial phase. You should check the rate every 6 months.

There are three methods to determine your HRmax:

1. **Performance diagnostics** is the safest method. Here, your lactate concentration is checked, or a respiratory gas analysis is carried out by a sports physician.

2. **You can use a formula.** However, I think this is too imprecise and too generalized. It is better to determine it actively, so I will not enter it here. When I use this formula, it shows me an HRmax that is about 10 bpm too high. This can have a negative effect on your training.

3. **The self-test.** It is best to go to a tartan track.
   Run in at your leisure (10–15 min).
   Then complete a 3 × 400 m or 3 × 300 m test program.
   1 × 400 m at a brisk pace
   2 min break
   1 × 400 m very fast
   2 min break
   1 × 400 m sprint at your limit
   Look at your heart rate monitor at the end and you will have determined your HRmax. But only if you have pushed yourself to the limit. Note that your heart rate may rise slightly approximately 10–20 seconds after the run. If it shows 192 bpm, for example, then round it up to 195, since most people are unable to push themselves to their absolute limit.

STRENGTH TRAINING

If we look at the requirements, it becomes clear that a pronounced strength-endurance training program is the most sensible way to make sure you pass the tests. As indicated above, mountains of muscle are rather counterproductive here.

However, if you have problems lifting the required weights often enough (beginners), I would recommend prior training to build muscle, as strength is a precondition. This maximum strength training can then be converted into targeted strength-endurance training. At least 6 months of muscle formation and 3–6 months of strength-endurance training would be advisable. I have always been a fan of high-quality training. And you cannot afford to waste time because the training workload is high. The "new wave" of calisthenics is also not suitable for recruitment tests. Do not get me wrong; the exercises are great and will complement any sport. I also like to incorporate them into my training—but not to prepare for tests like the bench press. You should prioritize conventional weight training until you are able to surpass the required performance by far. After that, you can incorporate sports such as CrossFit, Freeletics or Tabata training.

The problem is that many current training plans on the internet only consist of push-ups, squat jumps, burpees, and the like. Unfortunately, this is not effective. But remember: This statement does not apply to advanced-strength athletes. They will not suffer any disadvantages if they frequently perform their strength-endurance exercises. But I see time and time again that they are all able to do 50 push-ups, yet they have problems when they have to do 15 × 100 lb bench presses. But 100 lb is really not that much.

SWIM TRAINING

Regarding swimming, there are usually two distinct camps: swimmers and non-swimmers. I do not need to give swimmers advice or even write training plans for them. They will easily achieve the required times. To non-swimmers, I can only warmly recommend joining a swimming club for a short time. Because, apart from the training plans, the most important factor is training your technique. For this, a coach must stand at the edge of the pool and analyze your swimming style. The leg stroke, dipping of the hands, pulling and pushing, your position in the water, breathing, posture, and many more factors are of paramount importance. This is so complex that I cannot put it down in this paperback. There are, of course, countless YouTube videos which are supposed to show what to do. Beginners, however, are not able to implement these minute details. For athletes who are able to achieve a reasonably good time, I would still advise including swimming in their training plan. On the one hand, you will (re)gain a good sense of the water, which is essential for some tests (e.g., SEK, KSM). This is because combined underwater exercises are required, which means that you should feel at home in the water. On the other hand, swimming can also be put to good use to regenerate.

With two sessions per week, you will be able to (re)gain a sense of water. To achieve an increase in performance, I would recommend three sessions per week. I would advise an advanced swimmer not to waste too much time swimming, because swimming is often the "least important" part of the sports tests, and a good swimmer always passes it without any problems. A training session should consist of the warm-up, technique training, long or short sprint units, and the cool-down. You should train between for 45–60 minutes per session. You should alternate between long and short sessions and include apnea diving in your training.

Example:

Training day 1:
The long session: 6 × 500 m
500 m warm-up / 500 m technique / 500 m paddles / 500 m easy / 500 m fast / 500 m cool-down
Training day 2:
The sprints: 2,000–3,000 m
200 m warm-up / 200 m technique / 3 × 200 m progressive / 50 m easy / 4 × 100 m medley / 50 m easy / 6 × 50 m freestyle / 50 m easy / 6 × 50 m (25 m sprint with turnaround, 25 m easy back) / 50 m easy / 200 m cool-down

---

Sorry to let you down a little regarding swimming sessions. As already mentioned, swimmers do not need a plan; they know what they need to train for. However, a beginner needs to be assessed individually. This is why all-inclusive online plans are usually not very helpful. They either demand too much or too little from most people. I want to avoid this because I cannot promise you that an all-inclusive plan will actually help you. The best advice I can give you is to have an expert at hand, e.g., from a club or a friend who swims.

WARM-UP

Many athletes start their training without warming up. You can do this, but it is not advisable. The body compensates for a lot, sometimes for decades. But at some point, it's payback time if you have regularly stressed joints, ligaments, and muscles without warming up. The older you get, the more sensible an athlete you will become. Therefore, a short warm-up should precede every training session to prevent later wear and tear.

Running:

Here, I would briefly mobilize all the joints by rotating them. In addition, a run should always start with a warm-up. Start with 5–15 minutes before moving on to a harder main part.

Swimming:

Here, the shoulder muscles and joints cause problems. You can warm up before training by activating them with circular movements and always starting with a 200–400-meter swim. You can also use a rope to warm up gently.

Strength training:

A complex area, because here each muscle group/ joint is strained with additional weight. Depending on the type of training chosen, you can, for example, activate the rotator cuffs with elastic bands, start each strength unit with a light weight, or start with exercises using your own body weight.

STRETCHING

Hardly any other topic is as controversial as stretching. Sports scientists constantly bicker about the best stretching technique. Static or dynamic? Before training, or only afterward? Does stretching help at all? This is what sports magazine headlines will probably concern themselves with for decades to come.

But let's get down to the facts: In sports where speed is the main focus, stretching before training should be avoided. A sensible warm-up program makes much more sense here. Stretching can even lead to injuries in some areas. The situation is different again with sports such as martial arts. Maximum flexibility is required here, and stretching is therefore highly recommended.

What you do not achieve by stretching is protection against sore muscles. This has been proven scientifically. My personal approach to stretching: I have been an athlete for almost three decades. Starting with swimming, athletics, triathlon, and always strength training. I have hardly ever stretched in my life. Only when a trainer asked me to.

Did that do me any harm? Not in the first few years. At age 20, stretching sessions tend to be ridiculed. Even at age 30. When they pass 40, most athletes say: I wish I had stretched a bit more during my sports career.

Again, the problem is that a young body can cope with almost anything. However, the older you get, the more the disdain for stretching or fascia rolling takes its toll. Mobility suffers, and the muscles shorten. An athlete will only start stretching again after an injury and suddenly realize that it is really good for the body. I advise everyone to incorporate a short stretching session now and then. You can do this for 15 minutes, even in front of the television in the evening.

TRAINING DIARY

Training diaries are often scoffed at. But, especially in the age of tracking apps, it is easy to save and analyze the data recorded. You should do it too. But please collect everything in full and with a clear layout. There are ready-made files or apps on the internet. However, these are usually too generalized. You need a customized file. Of course, you can also use pencil and paper. But this is regularly too confusing. In an Excel spreadsheet, you can not only scroll quickly, but also view weekly or monthly summaries.

If you want to start a training diary, it should contain the following information: To provide a good overview, it should be kept on a weekly basis, with a short paragraph to provide you with an overview of all the kilometers and hours you have run during the week. Start with the date on the left. This is followed on the right by the training zone, e.g., BE1. In the next column, there is space for comments, e.g., intervals 4 × 1,000 m. Make columns for running, strength training, swimming, etc. Divide each of these into kilometers and time. For example, 10 km and 55 minutes. Then add the total training time if you complete several sessions per day. If you want to track your weight, you can add a column for weight and body fat at the end.

To make your work easier, we have created the *Fighting Fit Logbook,* which you can also purchase in the online shop.

COMPETITIONS

A competition is the best way to complete a tough training program. This is where you really push yourself to the limit because other people compete against you. Every competition, however, should overlap with the requirements. There is no point in running 3 km for months and then opting for a 10 km race. There should also be no further fast runs in the week of the competition.

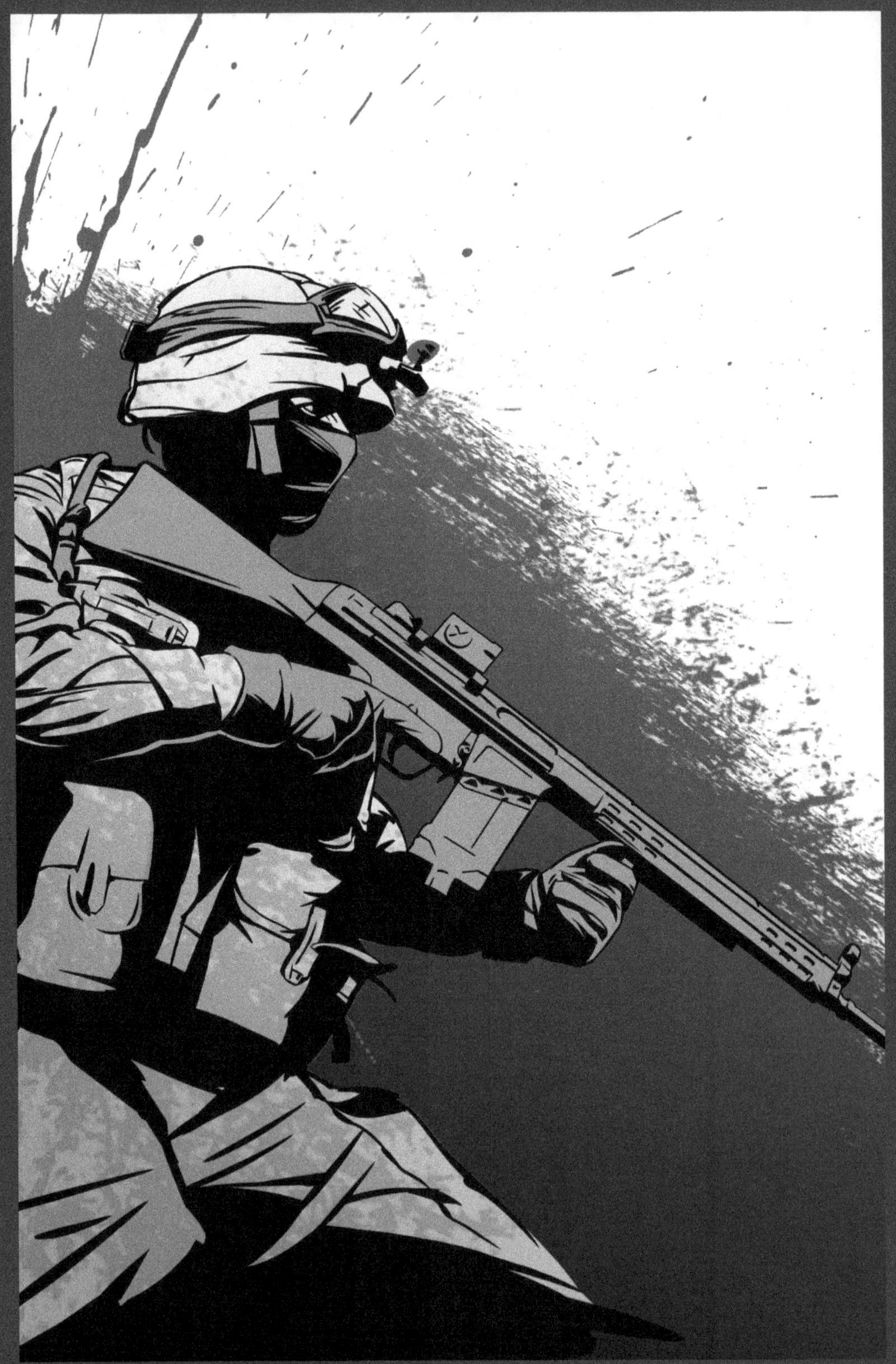

GENERAL TRAINING PLANS

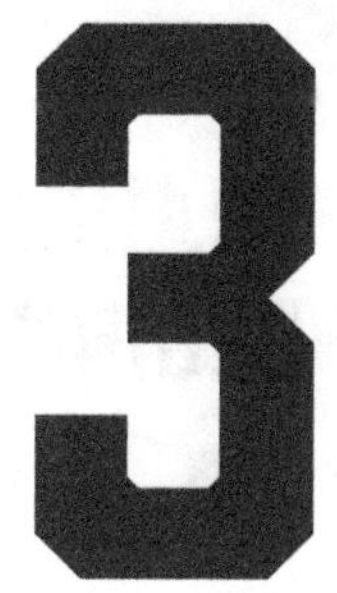

Key to the training plans

There are training zones in running that a runner who wants to achieve specific improvements needs to know. The following key is based on the maximum heart rate (HRmax).

Key:

RECOM	Recovery, HR in the lower range, up to 65 percent
BE1	Basic Endurance Zone 1, HR 65–80 percent (extensive = 60, intensive = 80 percent)
BE2	Basic Endurance Zone 2, HR (80–95 percent) (extensive = 80, intensive = 95 percent)
CSE	Competition-Specific Endurance, HR 995–100 percent
SERIES	A series consists of, e.g., 20–50 push-ups, sit-ups, and alternating jumps. Challenges every muscle group (biceps, triceps, chest, lower back, shoulders, abdomen, legs).
CIRCUIT TRAINING for STRENGTH	In the strength circuit, you initially train all muscle groups with one exercise. You alternate exercises with each workout. After a warm-up, you complete three rounds of 8–12 repeats.

TRAINING PLAN FOR BEGINNERS / 1 YEAR

WEEKS 1–3

In the first few weeks, we complete 2 running units, 2 strength-endurance units, and 2 swimming units. If you are already training for strength, train your specific workload. In the first week, do a 5 km run against the clock (at the limit) to get information on your progress.

Monday	–
Tuesday	running: 5 km test (at the limit), swimming
Wednesday	strength-endurance training 30 min (push-ups, squats, sit-ups, lower back)
Thursday	–
Friday	running 30 min BE1, swimming
Saturday	strength-endurance training 30 min (push-ups, squats, sit-ups, lower back)
Sunday	–

WEEKS 4–5

In these two weeks, we increase the number of running sessions to 3 and slightly increase the duration.

Monday	running: 35 min BE1
Tuesday	strength-endurance training 30 min (push-ups, squats, sit-ups, lower back)
Wednesday	running: 35 min BE1, swimming
Thursday	strength-endurance training 30 min (push-ups, squats, sit-ups, lower back)
Friday	–
Saturday	running: 35 min BE1, swimming
Sunday	–

WEEK 6

This is a RECOM week. We give the body the chance to regenerate so that it can really get going again in the following weeks.

Examples:

Mon–Sun	3 training sessions at will – but stick to a HR of 60–65 percent 1st training session: easy cycling for approx. 1 hour 2nd training session: easy strength-endurance training approx. 20–30 min or running 30 min 3rd training: swimming approx. 30–60 min

WEEKS 7–9

In these three weeks we increase the running distance and start with dumbbell exercises (never start circuit training with the same piece of gym equipment).

Monday	strength circuit
Tuesday	running 40 min BE1, swimming
Wednesday	–
Thursday	running 40 min BE1
Friday	strength circuit, swimming
Saturday	running 40 min BE1
Sunday	–

WEEK 10

RECOM week, as in week 6

WEEKS 11–13

In these three weeks, we again increase the running training but use 1 running session for active recovery. We therefore run within the extensive and intensive BE areas. And we add 1 strength unit to the training.

Monday	running 45 min BE1 int.
Tuesday	strength circuit, swimming
Wednesday	–
Thursday	running 30 min BE1 ext. / strength circuit
Friday	–
Saturday	running 45 min BE1 int., swimming
Sunday	strength circuit

WEEK 14

RECOM week, as in week 6

WEEKS 15–17

In these three weeks, we extend the running training into the BE2 zone. During strength training, we split up the different muscle groups.

Monday	running 40 min BE2, swimming
Tuesday	3 sets chest, 3 sets biceps, abs (warm up muscles before each exercise)
Wednesday	–
Thursday	running 40 min BE1 ext. / 3 sets of pull-ups 3 sets triceps, abs (warm up)
Friday	–
Saturday	running 50 min BE1 int., swimming
Sunday	150 push-ups (e.g., 5 × 30), 3 sets shoulder, abs? (warm up muscles before each exercise)

WEEK 18

RECOM week, as in week 6

WEEKS 19–21

As we have been dealing with zone BE2 over the past few weeks, we now increase the distance and extend the BE2 zone. Strength training remains at the usual level for the time being.

Monday	running 50 min BE2 int., swimming
Tuesday	3 sets chest, 3 sets biceps, abs (warm up the muscles before each exercise)
Wednesday	–
Thursday	running 40 min BE1 ext. / 3 sets pull-ups, 3 sets triceps, abs (warm up)
Friday	–
Saturday	running 60 min BE1 int., swimming
Sunday	150 push-ups (e.g., 5 × 30), 3 sets shoulder, abs (warm up muscles before each exercise)

WEEK 22

RECOM week, as in week 6

WEEKS 23–25

In these three weeks, we slowly move up from BE2 zone to the CSE zone. We vary strength training to provide the body with new stimuli. New series are added to slowly get accustomed to the training workload.

You can do interval training on the sports field (counting laps), but also on your running route by simply running on the basis of time spans. Examples of interval training on Saturdays:

Week 1:	warm-up 10 min / 3 × 800 m CSE with 3 min break / cool-down 10 min
Week 2:	warm-up 10 min 100 / 200 / 400 / 600 / 400 / 200 / 100 each with 2 min break / cool-down 10 min
Week 3:	warm-up 10 min / 30 × 20 s CSE with 30 s easy trot alternating / cool-down 10 min

Monday	running 10 min BE1, 40 min BE2, 10 min BE1
Tuesday	strength circuit, swimming
Wednesday	–
Thursday	running 45 min BE1 ext. / 5 × 20 series
Friday	–
Saturday	running 40 min CSE (interval training), swimming
Sunday	5 × 20 series, strength circuit

WEEK 26

RECOM week, as in week 6

WEEKS 27–29

Now that we have familiarised ourselves with interval training, we can increase it. We also increase the series.

Examples:

Week 1:	warm-up 10 min / 4 × 800 m CSE with 3 min break / cool-down 10 min
Week 2:	warm-up 10 min 100 / 200 / 400 / 600 / 400 / 200 / 100 each with 2 min break / cool-down 10 min
Week 3:	warm-up 10 min / 4 × 1,000 m CSE with 2–3 min break / cool-down 10 min

Monday	running 10 min, BE1, 40 min BE2 int., 10 min BE1 ext.
Tuesday	6 × 30 series, swimming
Wednesday	–
Thursday	running 45 min BE1 ext. / strength circuit
Friday	swimming
Saturday	running 40 min CSE (interval training)
Sunday	6 × 30 series

WEEK 30

RECOM week, as in week 6

WEEKS 31–33

Incorporate longer endurance runs. The interval training and BE2 training remain in place.

Monday	running 10 min BE1, 30 min BE2 int, 10 min BE1 ext.
Tuesday	6 × 40 series and strength training at will, swimming
Wednesday	–
Thursday	running: week 31: 70 min BE1 ext. week 32: 75 min week 33: 80 min
Friday	strength training at will (eliminate weaknesses), swimming
Saturday	running 40 min CSE (interval training)
Sunday	6 × 40 series

WEEKS 34–35

RECOM weeks; we take the time to slow our bodies down a little. The last three-week block was very intense. Therefore, we allow ourselves two weeks of active recovery. Schedule the following training as you wish:

1 × run 30 min (60–65 percent HRmax) on day 4
2 × swimming 30–45 min
2 × cycling 60 min
2 × series with light strength exercises at will

Recover properly during the breaks, and put your feet up for once!

WEEKS 36-38

In the next few weeks, the aim is to train away any remaining weaknesses, increase the duration of your easy runs, add a little more intensity to your interval training, and work through the series in a fun way.

Monday	running 10 min BE1, 40 min BE2 int., 5 min BE1 ext.
Tuesday	5 × 50 series, strength-endurance exercises at will
Wednesday	swimming
Thursday	running 80–90 min BE1 ext. / strength training at will (eliminate weaknesses)
Friday	–
Saturday	running 60 min CSE (interval training)
Sunday	5 × 50 series, swimming

WEEK 39

RECOM week, as in week 6

WEEKS 40–42

We have reached a good level and are trying to maintain it.

Monday	running 60 min BE2
Tuesday	series as you think fit or swimming
Wednesday	–
Thursday	running 80–90 min BE1 ext. / strength training at will (eliminate weaknesses)
Friday	–
Saturday	running 60 min CSE (interval training; train what you enjoy at even higher speed)
Sunday	series at will / swimming

WEEK 43

RECOM week, as in week 6

WEEKS 44–46

After we have been allowed to train as we please in the last few weeks, this is the week of the 5 km test (100 percent). Now you will see how much you have improved and whether it is enough to get you through the training. But I have no doubt about that.

Monday	running 10 min BE1, 45 min BE2 int., 5 min BE1 ext. / swimming
Tuesday	5 × 50 series
Wednesday	–
Thursday	running 80–90 min BE1 ext. / strength circuit
Friday	swimming
Saturday	running: 5 km test (100%)
Sunday	5 × 50 series

WEEK 47

RECOM week, as in week 6

WEEK 48

The last hard week before we rest and prepare for SOF training.

Monday	running 20 min BE1, 30 min BE2 int., 10 min BE1 ext.
Tuesday	50 series, as many as you can manage, in as short intervals as possible or swimming
Wednesday	–
Thursday	running 80–90 min BE1 ext. / strength circuit
Friday	–
Saturday	running 60 min CSE (interval training), swimming
Sunday	5 × 50 series

WEEKS 49–51

Before you start SOF training, it is important to wind down your body. Your body needs to regenerate completely. The training will be very exhausting and will push you to your physical and mental limits.

GOOD LUCK!

WHO DARES WINS

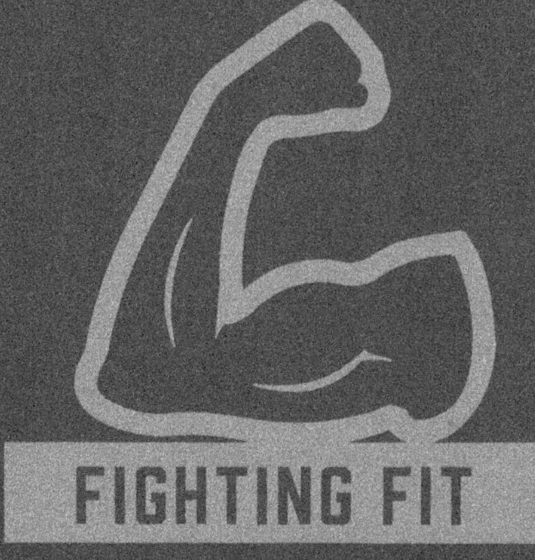

TRAINING PLAN FOR ADVANCED ATHLETES (6 MONTHS)

WEEKS 1–3

In the first three weeks, we want to get back into training and spend a maximum amount of time in the BE2 zone. We use the strength circuit for strength training so as not to overdo it at the beginning.

Monday	running BE2 ext. (10 min warm-up / 3 × 1,500 m BE2 with 500 m trot break / 10 min cool-down)
Tuesday	swimming, strength circuit
Wednesday	running 50 min BE1 (plus running ABC)
Thursday	–
Friday	strength circuit
Saturday	running 60 min BE1
Sunday	swimming, strength circuit

WEEK 4

This is a RECOM week. We allow the body to regenerate so that it can really get going again in the following weeks.

Mon–Sun	Do 3 training sessions at will, but stay below a HR of 65 percent. 1st training session: easy cycling for approx. 1 hour 2nd training session: easy strength-endurance training approx. 20–30 min or running 30 min 3rd training: swimming approx. 30–60 min

WEEKS 5–7

In these weeks, we will extend the BE2 zone a little and concentrate on muscle formation during strength training (3 months). You will therefore only train individual muscle groups during strength training.

Example:

Day 1:	chest / biceps / abdomen
Day 2:	back / triceps / lower back
Day 3:	shoulders / legs / abdomen
Monday	running BE2 int. (10 min warm-up/ 3 × 2,000 m GA2 with 500 m trot break / 10 min cool-down)
Tuesday	swimming
Wednesday	running 60 min BE1 (plus running ABC), strength training

Thursday	–
Friday	strength training
Saturday	running 70 min BE1, strength training
Sunday	swimming

WEEK 8

RECOM week, as in week 4

WEEKS 9–11

We keep up the muscle formation and increase our runs into the CSE range. You should do the interval training on the sports field.

Monday	running 40–50 min; interval training in the CSE zone
Tuesday	swimming, strength training
Wednesday	–
Thursday	running 50 min BE1 (plus running ABC), strength training
Friday	–
Saturday	running 60 min BE2, (10 min warm-up, 30–40 min BE2, 5–10 min cool-down)
Sunday	swimming, strength training

WEEK 12

RECOM week, as in week 4

WEEKS 13–15

In these weeks we add a 4th running session in the BE1 zone to muscle formation.

Monday	running 50–60 min; interval training in the CSE zone
Tuesday	swimming, strength training
Wednesday	running 50 min BE1 (plus running ABC), strength training
Thursday	–
Friday	running 60 min BE2, (10 min warm-up, 3 × 3,000 m BE2 with 500 m trot break, 5 min cool-down)
Saturday	swimming, strength training
Sunday	running 45 min BE1

WEEK 16

RECOM week, as in week 4

WEEKS 17-19

In these weeks, we move away from muscle formation and work on strength-endurance. We will also only do three runs per week and extend the BE1 runs slightly. You can find exercises for strength-endurance training in my book, Military Fitness. I will only list a few of the countless exercises available. But above all, you should practice more push-ups and pull-ups for your SOF training.

Example:

- total resistance exercise training
- kettle bell training
- body weight exercises, push-ups, pull-ups, partner exercises, etc.
- series (as described in the key)

Monday	interval training 60 min (week 17 BE2, week 18 BE2, week 19 CSE)
Tuesday	swimming, strength training
Wednesday	running 45 min BE1 (plus running ABC), strength training
Thursday	–
Friday	–
Saturday	swimming, strength training
Sunday	BE1 running: week 17: 70 min week 18: 80 min week 19: 90 min

WEEK 20

RECOM week as in week 4

WEEK 21

I leave the schedule for this week to you. Work on your weaknesses one last time. Continue to train in the BE1/2 and CSE zones. By now, you know best what is good for you and what will advance your fitness.

WEEKS 22-23

Done! You have reached the last two weeks before SOF training starts! Now it is extremely important that you give your body the rest it needs to recover. SOF training will be very exhausting and will push you to your physical and mental limits.

2 weeks	rest and easy cycling, easy swimming, easyrunning

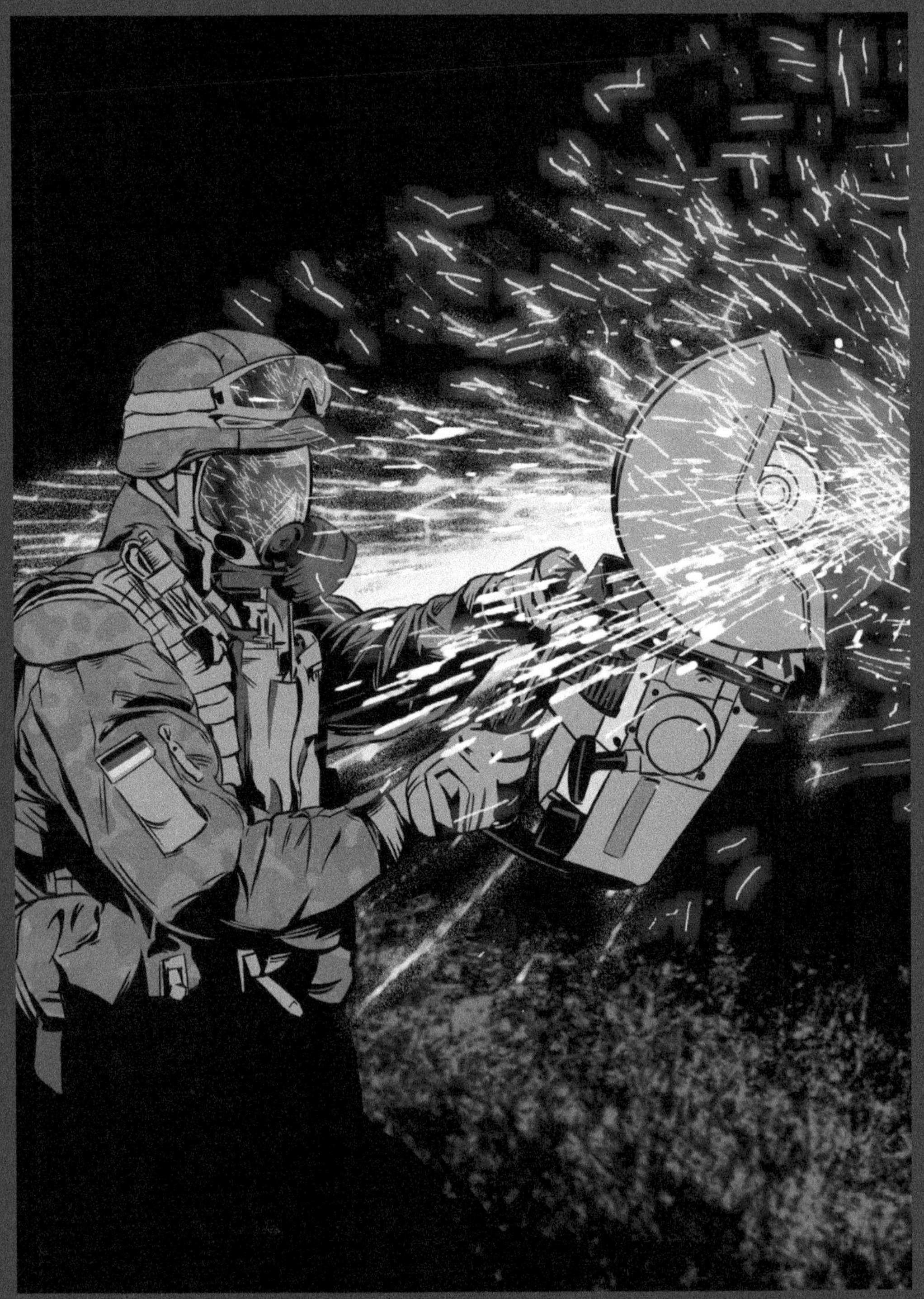

SPECIAL TRAINING PLANS

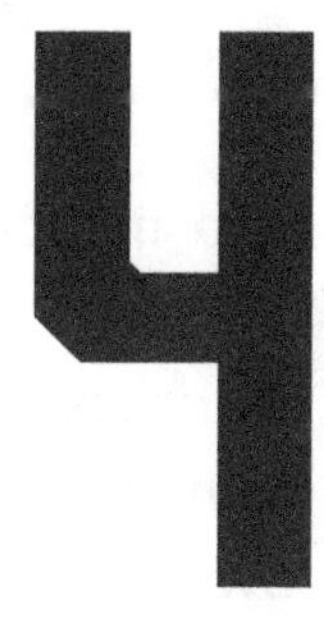

EXTREME SOF TRAINING MEANS EXTREME PREPARATION!

If you want to survive in an elite unit, you should be aware that your body and mind will be under maximum strain for a very long time. In the case of "Kampfschwimmer", for 7 months or even longer. Special preparation is required to master this challenge.

These tips are for athletes who not only focus on passing the entrance test, but also systematically prepare for the tough training period that follows.

For the last few weeks before SOF training, I advise advanced athletes to replace the interval units with a unit taken from the following routines.

The following training sessions do not come close to the workload you will face during SOF training. However, you can prepare your body for one or another strain. There will be no long breaks during SOF training. You will even be woken up at night to prove your mettle. During training, chafing and extremely sore muscles are no reasons to skip a sports session or miss a day. After a certain number of days' absence, you will be dropped from the training program. If you performed well enough, you may be allowed to repeat the program.

It is therefore advisable to get out of your comfort zone and push your body. But do not go to extremes, because the implementation of our training plan with its regeneration units makes perfect sense.

"NUMQUAM RETRO"

("Never back")
Motto of the Jagdkommando – Austrian Armed Forces Commandos

TIPS FOR THE PRO

▸ RUNNING WITH YOUR BOOTS ON, LOADS, IN WET CLOTHING, AND IN THE COLD

Complete a running session in hiking or combat boots, and you will see that the competitive runner suddenly finds it very difficult. This is because the running style is completely distorted. It is more like stomping than running in the midfoot or even forefoot area. The weight of the boot and its stiffness can become problematic.

▸ LOAD UP YOUR RUCKSACK

Grab a rucksack, fill it with about 10 kg of weight, and run a few kilometers. Use a material that completely fills the rucksack to prevent it from bouncing around.

▸ GET WET

Step briefly into a lake to get your boots completely wet, and you will see that it feels like you are dragging an anchor behind you. Add to the difficulty by getting into the water up to your belt in your military trousers. Not only will it feel heavier and more uncomfortable on your skin, but can also cause abrasions.

▸ MILITARY SWIM RUN

Please only do this with a training partner. Take a lake or a canal, for example. Complete your running lap, jump into the cool water again and again, and swim quickly for a few minutes. Then continue running. You can also do this in military trousers to make it even more difficult.

▸ CARRY YOUR COMRADE

Carrying comrades simulates a casualty-carrying exercise. Special forces worldwide, especially in the military, attach great importance to these exercises. After all, anyone who is unable to pull a wounded comrade out of the danger zone has no place in a special unit.

Go into the woods pairwise and take turns carrying each other. Uphill, downhill. You will realize that it is not just carrying that causes problems, but also being carried, because having a shoulder pushing into your stomach is not a nice feeling. Use different carrying methods: fireman's carry, pulling, dragging, the Rautek maneuver, etc.

▸ CARRY TREE TRUNKS OR LARGE STONES

You can simulate heavy equipment by carrying logs or stones. Simply take a large stone or tree trunk that you are barely able to carry and keep it with you for an hour while running or marching fast. Or repeatedly carry these items up and down a hill. Give yourself a short break and start again.

▸ RUN OFF-ROAD WITH STRENGTH UNITS

Do yourself a favor, and do not always run your familiar route. Take a turning and cross a field or run through the forest. You will often be moving off-track during your training.

▸ CAUTION! RISK OF INJURY FROM TWISTING AN ANKLE

The positive thing is that it toughens the small muscles and tendons. Always incorporate short strength training sessions into your running sessions. For example, warm up for 10 minutes and then start with 30 push-ups and 30 sit-ups. Every 5 minutes, incorporate other exercises, such as using bars for pull-ups. Do Spider-Man push-ups and practice jumps (e.g., frog jumps, calf jumps, alternating jumps, squat jumps, or squats), carry your training partner up a hill, or run 50 meters in duck walk, crab walk, or bear walk. Start running together. After 10 easy minutes, one of you does 20 push-ups and tries to catch up with the other. Of course, the other person continues to run at a relaxed pace. Repeat this routine as often as you like.

▸ MARCHES WITH HEAVY LOADS

In the military, marches are simply part of the game. In the special forces, you not only have to march, but also carry a lot of special equipment with you, which means that your rucksack is bound to be very heavy. Weights in excess of 50 kg are not uncommon.

But you should take care of your back so that you can start your SOF training fresh and uninjured. Therefore, simply take a weight that you consider to be heavy (e.g., 20–30 kg), put on your hiking boots, and walk for 2–3 hours at a brisk pace.

SPECIAL ADVICE REGARDING THE UNITS

▶ ADDITIONAL TRAINING KSM [GERMAN NAVY SEALS]

During your training to become a "Kampfschwimmer", you will have to complete one or a number of series almost every day. A series consists of push-ups, sit-ups, and and alternating jumps, or alternatively: squats or lying down/standing up. It all starts in the first week with a series of 20. This means that a series is only declared complete when the entire class has completed 20 push-ups, sit-ups, and alternating jumps at the same time. Ten repetitions are added every week, so that you reach the 50 series in 4 weeks. This will be maintained for the rest of the training period.

Be careful, however! If there are any inconsistencies or breaks during a series, the instructor may well start a series from scratch again. Make sure you train the 50 series in one go. Even several times in a row.

It is advisable to do an internship at the KSM beforehand. You can get information from the Personalwerbetrupp (PWT, Personnel Recruitment Office), **find contact details at the end of the book.**

▸ ADDITIONAL TRAINING KOMMANDO SPEZIALKRÄFTE (KSK) – GERMAN SPECIAL FORCES COMMAND

The crucial point is “Hell Week.” March until you are completely exhausted and yet be fit enough in your head to fulfill all the tasks that await you. The **Tips for the Pro** will help you with this.

Here, the motto is to go beyond your limits. You should complete a good mix of marches and runs during preparation. But do not overdo it with the marches. A few weeks beforehand is enough, as the risk of overstraining yourself by marching for hours and further training is extremely high. The aim should be to get your tendons and muscles used to boots and luggage. The most difficult part, which you should not underestimate, is the Aptitude Assessment Procedure 1. They test your knowledge in all areas. From computer tests to interviews by psychologists and memorization tasks. You should prepare for this conscientiously.

▸ ADDITIONAL TRAINING SEK (SPECIAL TASK FORCES OF THE GERMAN POLICE)

The SEK has differing requirements, depending on the federal state. In Schleswig-Holstein, for example, there is a small self-defense scenario with the aim of showing that you are able to defend yourself in a boxing match. No trained boxer is required here. This is a test of stamina, willpower, and courage. It does not hurt to put on your boxing gloves from time to time. Because if you have never taken a punch to the head, you will be surprised.

▸ ADDITIONAL TRAINING GSG 9

In contrast to the military units, there is a commission in the GSG 9 which asks specific questions to assess a candidate's character. But you also have the opportunity to introduce and “sell” yourself the best you can. You should therefore inform yourself properly in advance, weigh up the pros and cons, and not just take the test for fun.

You may be thinking: What a load of rubbish! If you apply for a commando job, you must have done all the research beforehand and want to do this job with your heart and soul. Far from it! I have met good athletes who just wanted to give it a go. Without the necessary expertise. Without knowing what was in store for them. That finished them off relatively quickly. **So, do it right or do not do it at all!**

▸ ADDITIONAL TRAINING AUSTRIAN COMMANDOS

Push-ups. Running. Pull-ups. At the end of the day, what counts is that you have to be a tenacious, tough machine. Regardless of whether you are faced with a forced backpack march or just several push-ups. Strength and endurance are the keys to remaining cognitively resilient while being completely stressed out.

LEARN TO SUFFER PAIN WITHOUT COMPLAINING

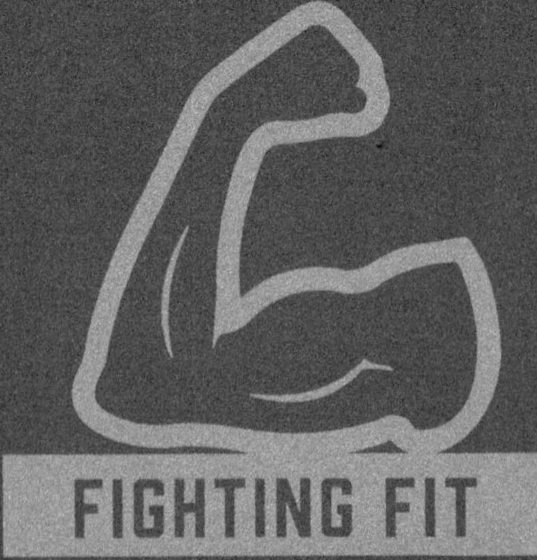

NUTRITION

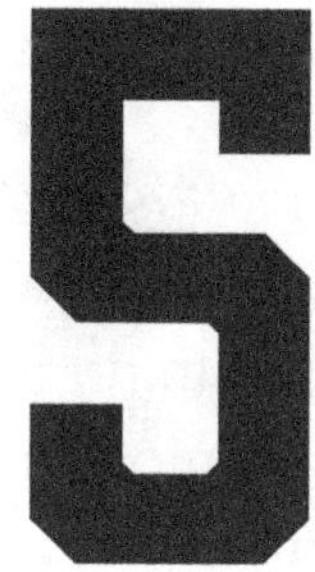

NUTRITION PLAYS AN ESSENTIAL ROLE IN EVERY ATHLETE'S PREPARATION FOR A COMPETITION.

Be it in the regeneration phase or shortly before a competition, as you are preparing for an important stage in your life, SOF training can be seen as a kind of competition. Because the journey is so short, you will wish you had had three or four more months to prepare. Nutrition fills entire books, so there is no way I can cover everything here. However, I would like to emphasize that a one-sided diet will lead to a drop in performance, and you will not be able to achieve your personal maximum despite a tough training plan.

A focused diet makes the body more efficient. It will be able to regenerate better and build up muscle. The risk of injury is reduced, and the body is better able to cope with setbacks. Alongside interval units, regeneration is the most important component of training. If you train hard, you need to regenerate. I achieve this through a well-organized training plan on the one hand and nutrition on the other. One keyword here is the open-window effect.

Everyone should be aware that one-sided diets are harmful. A balanced diet provides the body with everything it needs to be, and remain, efficient. In my opinion, a sophisticated nutrition program is something for top athletes. Because this is where seconds can be gained. But is that relevant to us? Probably not. So eat sensibly and do not drive yourself crazy. Do not think about your diet all day long. Listen to your body, it will tell you what it needs. However, if you need to lose weight, other principles apply. Read more about this under Diets.

▶ FOOD SUPPLEMENTS

I would avoid taking too many supplements. Because if you make your body dependent on various "permitted" substances, you may suffer a drop in performance if you are suddenly no longer able to use these substances. The standard products that can be found in many cupboards are: BCAA, amino acids, whey protein, hard gainers, protein shakes, vitamins, Frubiase, L-arginine, etc.

That is all well and good. You can also find most of this in a balanced diet.

But to do this, you need to take a sensible approach to the subject. In my years as a competitive athlete, I took protein supplements and omega-3 capsules. I got my carbohydrates in the form of pasta or potatoes. All other important nutrients can be found in a balanced diet.

Beer, wine, chocolate, and other sweets are, of course, allowed from time to time. After all, hard sporting preparation shapes the body all by itself. You should therefore treat yourself from time to time.

However, if you still need to work on your performance and want to tease out the last nuances by means of your diet, I recommend that you do so without those treats. In this case, you should get tips from a good nutritionist.

▶ DIETS

Why am I talking about diets separately here? This topic is very important because you should not be on a diet while preparing intensively. Cutting out important parts of nutrition, such as in the low-carb diet, means that your body does not have the energy it needs for hard interval units. If you were to train hard, your body would not be able to realize 100 percent of your training. Of course, you will get better, but you will be wasting time because you could do it much more effectively. This does not apply to athletes who have permanently changed their diet. Athletes who have been eating this way for years have adjusted their bodies to it.

The best thing to do is to set aside enough time to diet and do a light fat-burning workout beforehand until you have reached your target weight (2–4 months).

After that, you can switch to a normal diet and concentrate fully on your training sessions.

Example:

Months	1–3: fat-burning training and diet
Months	4–5: intensified training sessions, longer and slightly harder runs, and a normal diet
Months	6–12: precise interval training and exercises at the limit, paired/coupled with regeneration units and an adapted diet. Your food intake will usually be significantly higher in this phase, as you burn a lot of calories during the hard and frequent sessions

When losing weight, it is important not to use the proverbial crowbar. It is best to lose 2–5 kg per month to achieve long-term success and thus avoid a yo-yo effect.

▸ WEIGHT GAIN

For very lean athletes with a high metabolism, it is advisable to build up mass. In the course of SOF training, the body loses substance. This can be especially critical for lean athletes, as they can become more susceptible to illness and injury. This is also an exclusion criterion for some units. After all, if you are frequently ill or injured, you cannot be relied on during routine duty, let alone during operations.

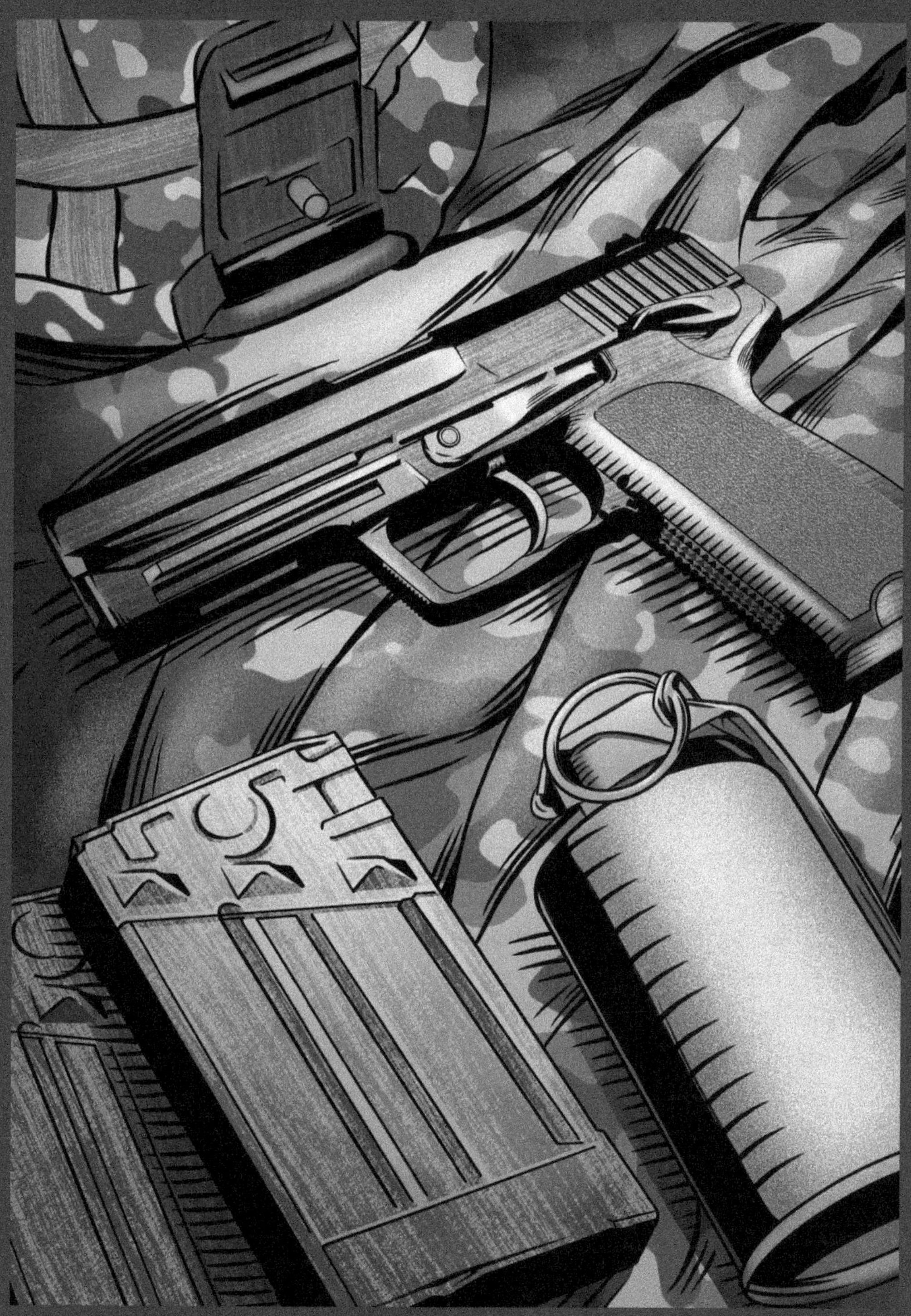

MENTAL STRENGTH

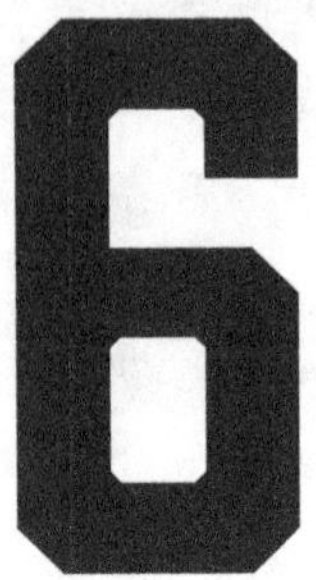

IT IS SAID THAT THE EXTRA MILE IS BETWEEN YOUR EARS. HOW TRUE!

During my time as a “Kampfschwimmer” recruit, I learned that the longer the course went on, the more my mental ability developed. The physical demands were, of course, brutal. But motivating yourself again and again is a massive mental challenge. Unfortunately, many recruits fail for precisely this reason.

Once the initial test has been passed, the stress usually starts right away. The demands are increased, and the body must suffer. But mental strength is what keeps you going. It is not just the extreme situations, such as confined spaces, apnea diving, or high altitudes, that make your head spin. For some, the presence of a particular instructor or the fear of failure is enough.

It is your will that gets you across the finishing line. And to be honest, a bit of luck here and there. There are plenty of books on the subject of mental strength. Of course, you can also train your mental strength. But how do you become mentally strong?

It is a process that needs to develop. A strong team with whom you share the rigors of training is particularly helpful here. I have experienced this myself, which is why I would like to take this opportunity to thank the 2003 "Kampfschwimmer" training course once again.

The more difficult situations you master, the stronger you become. Your self-confidence increases, and you develop a kind of positive "don't give a shit" attitude. This attitude helps you overcome ordeals that are deliberately created by the instructors to push you to the limit. This does not mean that you should not care about anything. On the contrary. In training, however, it is a positive quality. You switch off and only work through the tests set for you. For as long as it takes, and even longer if necessary.

If you now think that you can learn this skill, I am sorry to say that not everyone is able to clear their head and become mentally strong enough to join an elite squad. There are people who read ten books on mental strength and still do not make it. There are, however, also helpful tips which (can) make the journey a little easier. In addition, theoretical knowledge cannot be tested, because you can only call on this strength in extreme situations. And these cannot be simulated in everyday life.

In the past, there was almost no information on the subject of special forces. Nevertheless, men with a strong will, the courage, and the drive to belong made it. Nowadays, we are literally inundated with information. But do we have more personnel in the special forces? Not really.

Although the entry requirements have been lowered, there has been only a slight increase. Although the number of applicants has increased, the quality has deteriorated. Many leave the training center very quickly.

My conclusion is that if you put your heart and soul into it, if you do not lose sight of your goal and are physically well-prepared, you have a realistic chance of completing the training program.

„FACIT OMNIA VOLUNTAS“

("The will decides")
Motto of the KSK

TRAINING AIDS

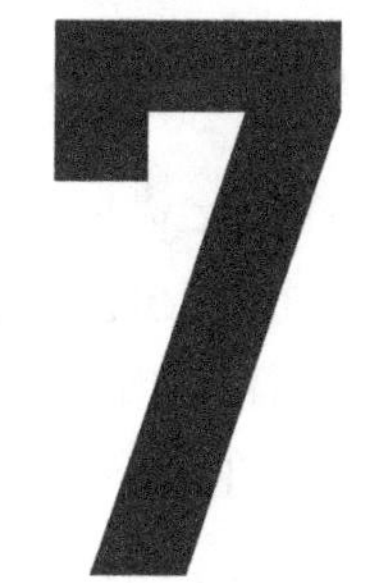

EVERYONE IS TALKING ABOUT TRAINING AIDS.

Even discount supermarkets have jumped on this bandwagon. CrossFit and the like use all kinds of equipment to make training more interesting. In my book, *Military Fitness,* I talk specifically about sling trainers and kettlebells. I even use a variety of training aids in my sports group.

But are these training aids useful to prepare for SOF training? I cannot answer this question with a clear yes or no. Let's s take a look at a few devices:

- **skipping rope**
- **sandbag/weight bag**
- **car tyres, tractor tyres**
- **push-up handles**
- **training mask**
- **kettlebell**
- **sling trainer**
- **exercise mat**
- **coordination ladder**
- **hurdles**
- **training rope/ battle rope**
- **weight vest/ plate carrier**

First, you have to ask yourself: What do I want to achieve? The answer is quite simple. You want to pass a test that consists of specific disciplines. If you already know that you can easily pass it, the next question is: What can you expect after the test? Are you sufficiently prepared for this?

These areas need to be trained specifically. So, if you are preparing for bench presses, why should you train with the battle rope?

Beginners who have massive problems with running and strength training should stay away from the wide range of equipment. This is because beginners have so much basic training to complete in their training plan that additional training with training aids would simply be too much. Their bodies would be overtaxed, and they would probably very soon become overtrained. Or they might not manage to reach the minimum requirements because they have done too much "unnecessary" training.

There are always people who ask me for a training plan but are not prepared to give up their "favorite hobby" for it.

FOR EXAMPLE:

An averagely trained man enjoys CrossFit. However, the training schedule I developed for him is so comprehensive that additional CrossFit training (2–3 times a week) would force him into overtraining, or he would neglect other more important units. This is because his deficits in individual disciplines are so great that he has no time for further training sessions. The regeneration phases would be too short.

However, he does not want to do without CrossFit because he believes that it can be combined well with other activities. In this example, the negative effects are that the legs are put under a lot of strain. With constantly sore muscles several times a week, a structured running training plan cannot be implemented properly. He tried it anyway and, after 6 months, confirmed my fears.

Trust what your trainers say, because they often have years of experience. Otherwise, you just waste time you frequently do not have!

It is difficult to achieve your goal with such an attitude. Unless you allow for a very long period of time, which is often not the case. Enjoying sports is important, but you can have fun again after your SOF training. If you have deficits, then focus your training on these gaps.

Most of the time, when I discuss the training plans, I already know who is passionate enough and would be able to master the requirements.

Advanced athletes can certainly use one or two training aids to push individual areas. For example, they can incorporate jump training with hurdles into their running training or make push-up training more difficult by using push-up grips.

Nevertheless, the motto also applies here: first the basics and targeted training sessions before other additional training is incorporated.

Pros should definitely incorporate training aids into their training. For them, it is no longer about improving their 5-km time even further or pushing 100 pounds even more often. They should become even more comprehensive athletes by additionally training intermediate and small muscles. Balance, coordination, and flexibility are also important factors. They also protect the body from injury.

HOW CAN I USE TRAINING AIDS IN A TARGETED WAY?

The **skippin rope** is a good full-body training tool. It strengthens the leg muscles (especially the calves), abdomen, lower back, and shoulders in the strength-endurance area. You can also compose very pleasant training sessions. Example: 10 × 30-second jumps with 10 push-ups in between (different variations).

I have already mentioned the **sandbag** (weight bag) in my book, *Military Fitness*. Various strength units can also be combined here. Depending on the weight, it is even possible to build up muscles. In addition to leg exercises (squats, lunges, etc.), you can also include the upper body. Although the upper body is permanently involved as it has to hold the bag. Biceps, triceps, etc. can be trained separately with targeted exercises.

A **car tire** (small) is ideal for hurling, throwing, holding, carrying, or pulling. Fitted with a rope, it becomes an additional weight for sprint units. A tractor tire can be worked on with a gym hammer or flipped over.

The **push-up handles** ensure that you get down even closer to the floor. This strains your chest muscle a little more and is therefore much more strenuous. On top of this, you can also incorporate movement games by using only one handle and remaining flexible when performing the push-ups.

The **training mask,** or altitude-training mask, cannot simulate altitude training. From a technical point of view, this is not possible. I do not believe in this mask at all, because tests have not shown any changes in the following areas:

- **oxygen intake**
- **aerobic and anaerobic capacity**
- **respiratory muscles**
- **lung function**
- **fatigue duration**
- **haemoglobin/haematocrit level**

Some results even turned negative. There are, however, two aspects that have changed positively, the ventilatory threshold and respiratory compensation. As the negative aspects predominate, this mask is, in my opinion, completely superfluous for training. What is more, it is outrageously expensive. You should concentrate on the basics and not follow every trend, unless you want to walk around the gym like Bane from *The Dark Knight Rises* and find yourself the object of derision.

The **kettlebell** is a piece of equipment that has been around for many years. I have also included this training in my book. Training with kettlebells is a workout for entire muscle groups. Depending on the weight, I can train in a variety of ways. Functional strength, explosive strength, and stability are required here.

Sling trainers are also included in the book, *Military Fitness*. There are over 300 exercises. Whether leg strength, upper body, full body, or combined training, everything is possible. But be careful; most of the exercises are in the strength-endurance range. So make sure you know what your goal is. There are inexpensive products that can easily compete with the overpriced branded products.

The **exercise mat**. Why is this on the list? Sure, you can lie on it. It is nice and soft. Training on it is very comfortable. But be careful! In almost all units, training sessions and tests will take place on the floor. Especially during SOF training. Do not get too comfortable, and leave your comfort zone from time to time. Because during SOF training, it is fatal if you get chafing on your back just because you have always made yourself too comfortable. Forget the mats for a while to see how uncomfortable some exercises can be on a hard floor.

The **coordination ladder** is ideal to train coordination. Not a must, but a welcome change to get out of the dreary training routine.

Hurdles are great training aids to practice all kinds of jumps. The jumps I would incorporate into your training every week will give you an immense increase in strength in your leg and gluteal muscles, which will not only benefit you when running.

Training ropes/battle ropes are now available in almost every gym. However, these are often not suitable, as I have seen thin, short ropes that are barely sufficient for a normally trained man to train effectively. There are different lengths and diameters. If you have already built up strength, I would recommend a 15-meter-long and 5-cm-thick rope. With this, units of 20–60 seconds are possible, depending on the exercise.

The **weight vest** is available in many versions. There are also military plate carriers for CrossFit training. Very comfortable to wear. But expensive, as the weights are often not included in the price.

Please be careful when running with weights. If you want to train to prepare for backpack runs, you should already be a good runner with good leg muscles. The weights are so hard on the joints that I would not recommend it when preparing for the recruitment test, except for the test at the KSK. Here, it is essential to prepare with a rucksack. But it is also best to wear boots and march. Fast-tempo runs with a rucksack are more in the 3-kilometer range, so you do not need to train specifically for this.

Running shoes are a big topic. But they are also big business.

As a triathlete (for over 23 years), I have worn out a few dozens of running shoes and have had a few painful experiences due to the wrong choice of shoes. The wrong shoes are sometimes the cause of problems with the knees, shins, or hips. But if you think that changing your running shoes is enough, you will soon be proven wrong. The main reason for injuries is too much strain due to training too hard or too long. You will have to push your body beyond normal limits when training for a special task force. Therefore, look out for early signs to prevent serious injury in good time. Because such an injury can mean the end, at least for the time being.

That would put your next opportunity to take part in a test a long way off.

It is a fact that around 85 percent of all runners require normal shoes. They should fit and be comfortable. Such shoes do not have to cost a lot of money. Until a few years ago, shoes with supports were popular, for example Duomax from Asics. Almost all manufacturers have moved away from this technology, as findings have shown that inward rolling is tolerable for most people and does not require additional support. Only 15 percent of runners need precisely adapted footwear. In this case, you should have a proper treadmill analysis carried out. But please not in a sports shop with poorly trained staff. An incorrect interpretation of the analysis will inevitably lead to pain and, therefore, long breaks in training.

If you train every day, it is best to alternate between two pairs of running shoes so that the cushioning of one pair can regenerate while the other is in use.

Heart rate monitors have become an indispensable part of everyday training. They are easily available. With standard basic functions, but also with functions which could not be more unnecessary. Is a heart rate monitor useful for my training?

Heart rate monitors are essential, especially for beginners. Almost all training plans are based on the individual heart rate. Beginners, but also good amateur runners, often do not know which training zone they are currently in. To make training as effective as possible, it is particularly important to know one's current heart rate zone. But does it have to be a luxury product? Absolutely not! Nevertheless, simple watches are, of course, very limited in their functions. They often lack a GPS function and a connection to the computer to download your running statistics. A watch in the medium price range offers everything beginners need to optimize training. For example, the Polar M430 or an equivalent from Garmin.

A GPS function should always be included. This guarantees the exact pace you are running at. Of course, every heart rate monitor covers your heart rate. The differences here lie in accuracy and transmission. In this case, you could almost say, the more expensive, the better.

For statistics freaks, it is also a nice gimmick to have the running routes displayed via maps and all possible details of the run. There are even training plans provided by the individual providers. A friend of mine trains according to such a plan, and we have found out that it is hardly any different from my old system. Which, of course, I think is a good endorsement of my approach. The good models are also quite stylish, so you can also wear a good sports watch as an everyday watch.

Is a **chest strap** absolutely necessary? Everyone is moaning about the chest strap. I can well understand that. It slips and is annoying at first due to the oppressive feeling it creates. The watch, however, measures your pulse while you are wearing it on your wrist. This function is rather unreliable for active sports such as jogging. On the bike, however, the readings are transmitted very accurately. Especially in winter, there are always inaccuracies that lead to athletes training in the wrong training zone. That is why I always recommend wearing a chest strap. Of course, it costs a little money at the beginning. But it is worth it, as it also transmits other readings, such as ground contact time, etc.

TRAINING MYTHS

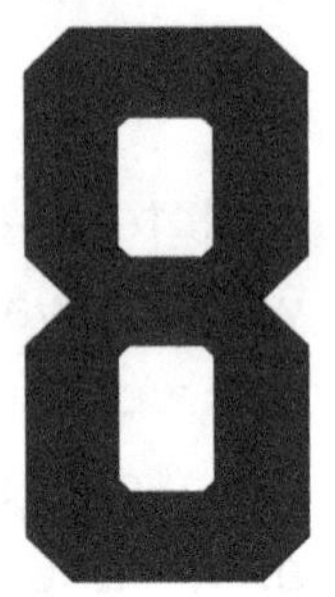

GOOGLE "TRAINING MYTHS" AND YOU WILL BE FACED WITH AN ABUNDANCE OF EXAMPLES, MOST OF THEM IRRELEVANT.

I have picked out a few that are important for us.

1. NO PAIN, NO GAIN

Anyone who has read and understood this book will realize that this is complete bunk. Because a lasting and healthy increase in performance can only be achieved if the hard units are balanced with regeneration units.

2. ALWAYS STRETCH BEFORE YOU TRAIN

The aim of stretching is to reduce basic tension in the muscles, loosen them up a little and make them more supple. But the exact opposite is the case, because the muscle reacts to stretching by contracting. This is not conducive to the upcoming training sessions. It is better to warm up specifically for the sports session. For strength training, exercises with light weights are sufficient beforehand; for running, I would recommend a 2-minute mobilization program and a relaxed warm-up run of 10 minutes.

3. FAT ONLY GETS BURNED AFTER 30 MINUTES

This myth should not really concern us during preparations for an elite unit test. I only consider a 30-minute workout when I am short on time or in the regeneration phase. But this statement is interesting because it has been around for decades. It is a fact that fat is burned right from the start. Sometimes a little faster and sometimes a little slower, depending on the intensity of the session. However, once the carbohydrate storage is empty, prepare for a bonfire of fat.

4. REGULAR JOGGING IS BAD FOR YOUR JOINTS

If there are no injuries, you are not very overweight, and you wear sensible shoes, regular jogging is actually beneficial. Cartilages need to be strained and relaxed, which is the case when jogging. So get out into nature.

5. MUSCLES MAKE THE BODY IMMOBILE

Normal muscle growth improves mobility. However, if you do not train the antagonist muscles properly, this can quickly lead to problems. It should also be clear that we are not talking about bodybuilding here, where movement restrictions due to acquired muscle mass are part of the game.

6. IF YOU SWEAT A LOT, YOUR PHYSICAL CONDITION IS POOR

This topic cannot be generalized in any way. There are differences in sweating. On the one hand, an athlete can have significantly more sweat glands and therefore sweat much more than another athlete at the same level of performance. This is not an indicator of poorer fitness. On the other hand, there are well-trained athletes who sweat a lot, but whose sweat consists mainly of water and not electrolytes. You can often see this in their clothing. If there is a high loss of electrolytes, white edges form around the sweat stain. Sweat formation in very overweight people is a completely different issue.

7. EXERCISING ONCE A WEEK IS NOT WORTH IT

A much-discussed but inaccurate view in the event of injury, illness, or lack of time. Because it is better to train once than not at all! If you can manage only one session per week due to time constraints, you should do maximum strength training. If you know in advance that you will not have time in a particular week, then make it a recovery week. For the average athlete, every training session makes sense, even if it is only once a week. But there is no way we can be satisfied with such a time allotment for preparation purposes.

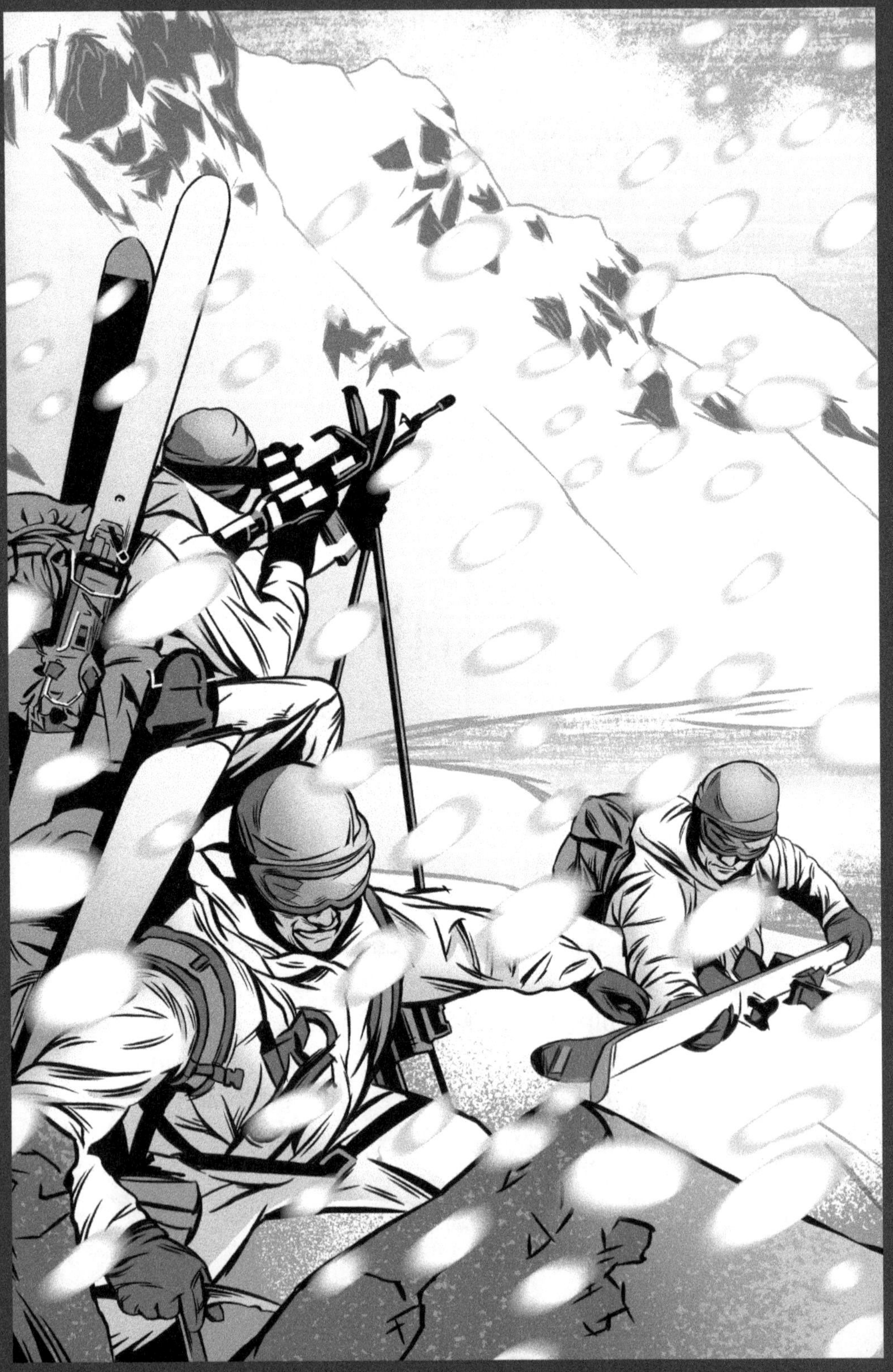

FAQ & IMPORTANT ISSUES

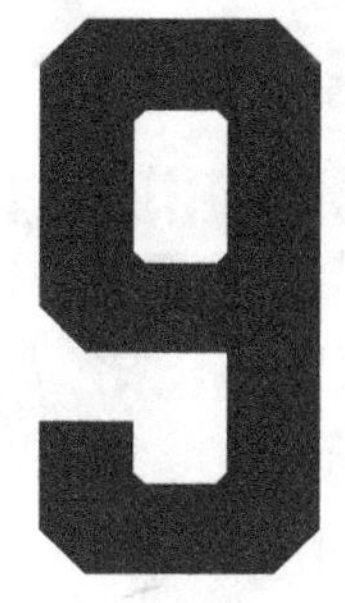

HOW EARLY DO I NEED TO START WITH TARGETED TRAINING?

That depends on your level of performance. But in my experience, starting training 4 months in advance is too short. I would allot 6–9 months for advanced athletes and at least a year for beginners (see Chapter 2).

CAN I APPLY TO AN ELITE UNIT AT THE AGE OF 17?

Of course, there are comrades who have started and completed their training at such a young age. But this is the exception rather than the rule. Candidates who fail at such a young age often do not come back. That is a shame, because many of them have potential. Give yourself enough time to train and deal with the issue in a targeted manner. Find out about the recruitment requirements of the units in question, because they differ.

I WOULD LIKE TO GIVE IT A GO, BUT I THINK I AM TOO UNATHLETIC. IS THERE ANY WAY I CAN TEST MYSELF?

That is easy; just read the minimum requirements for the unit in question and take the tests. If you can do them, complete them in one day. If you are good enough, your next step should be an application and focused training.

WHICH IS MORE IMPORTANT? STRENGTH OR ENDURANCE?

As you can see from the various chapters, it is mainly strength-endurance training that is required, although strength is definitely included. Do not confuse muscle mass with strength. You do not have to aim for a 18-inch upper arm to have enough strength. Your goal should be a perfect mix of endurance in running and strength in the strength tests.

CAN ANYONE HELP ME WITH MY PREPARATION? ARE THERE ANY TRAINING GROUPS?

It depends on your personal fitness. I have managed without any training groups or help. But I have been doing sports for over 20 years. If you have deficits in swimming, you should join a swimming club for a short period of time. There are trainers there who can specifically address your problems. A gym membership would be sensible if you have no other way of doing accurate strength training. When running, it is enough if you can motivate yourself well and follow my training guidelines. However, a training partner is always helpful, and it is also more fun with a partner. There are also running groups or running clubs in almost every city that you can join.

THREE IMPORTANT THINGS TO BEAR IN MIND DURING PREPARATION:

DO NOT LOSE SIGHT OF YOUR GOAL

There will be situations during your preparation that will set you back. Even if it is only by a week or two. For example, illness, an accident, changes at work, or personal problems. In this case, it is important to keep calm. You have already put your body under a lot of strain. It will not immediately lose the fitness it has built up. Admittedly, restarting is tough. Your legs are heavy, and your heart rate is unusually high. But after a short period of familiarisation, you will be back on track.

DO NOT TAKE THE PREPARATION LIGHTLY

At the beginning, the goal is still a long way off. Your training has not really picked up speed yet, and you are taking your time. That is a mistake. Because the closer the deadline gets, the more often you critically look at your times and repetitions. Suddenly, you realize that it is not quite enough yet, and you start to get nervous. Now you take out the crowbar. That will not work. The earlier you train, the more confidence you will have just before the tests and SOF training.

STICK TO THE PLAN

Once you have decided on a training plan, stick to it. Do not jump back and forth; be patient, because all good training plans are structured. Sometimes you only see the results after a few weeks. The body tends to stagnate, especially over a period of 3–4 months, and you think you have to change something. But that is normal. Now it is time to stick with it and keep going. Never believe promises made on the internet. Nobody will get you in top shape in just a few weeks.

CLOSING REMARKS

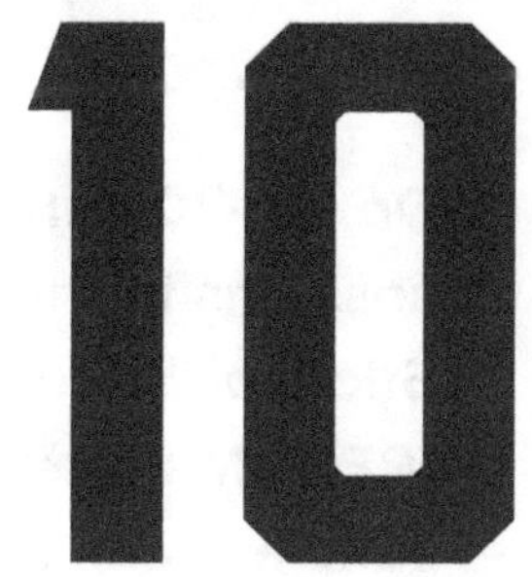

I AM A FRIEND OF TARGETED TRAINING METHODS.

Social networks are full of novelties and tips. Everyone wants to sell something. Sometimes the old concepts are portrayed as bad and outdated, and scientific-sounding theories are spouted that no normal person understands. Do not let this confuse you.

I tested some of this stuff on my former Facebook page "Military Fitness/Schreiber/Aumann" for quite a while. Not everything on the market is bad. But think carefully about whether it will help your training or just waste your time during the preparation phase. Do not spend too much time unnecessarily on fancy stuff. Because the sports that are required are centuries old. All you have to do is train them. Pay attention to the following items, and you will be successful in the long term:

- **Do 60–70 percent of your running sessions in the Basic Endurance Zone 1 (BE1).**
- **Stick to the regeneration phases (RECOM units).**
- **Take a break if you fall ill to avoid making the illness worse.**
- **Allow enough time for preparation.**
- **If possible, train with a training partner or coach.**

GOING BACK TO THE ROOTS IS THE KEY TO SUCCESS. FOCUS ON THE ESSENTIALS.

If there is enough time to do other sports or use sports equipment, I am the last person to object, because training with training aids is fun and can be useful.

But first, you have to get the basics right. And these are almost always running, strength training, and swimming. Everything else is secondary. There are also many books that want to show you how to become an elite soldier or a perfect athlete.

Sure, that can work. But the publishers of these books are often people who have trained for years to be as fit as they are today. So be clever, take what you need from the books, and incorporate this into your training. But remember, no one has ever become a world champion just by reading. You can find useful book tips in Chapter 12.

It is not necessary to be a top athlete. Good fitness, coupled with an iron will, is the key to success. Trust your abilities and try to be among the best everywhere.

THE WILL DECIDES

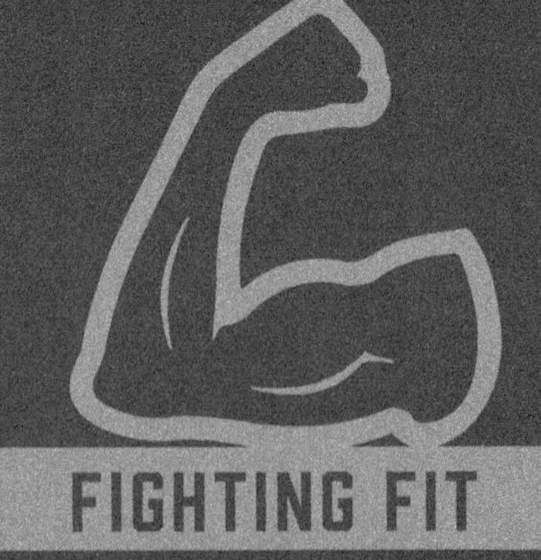

REQUIRE-MENTS

11

ALL UNITS HAVE ONE THING IN COMMON: THEIR SPECIFIED ENTRY REQUIREMENTS ARE MINIMUM REQUIREMENTS.

If you barely pass the entry-level test, you can be sure that your training path will end after a few days. This is because demands increase dramatically. Everyone should therefore endeavor to exceed these minimum requirements many times over. Running and strength exercises are the basic variables in the tests for all units. Swimming also often enters the mix.

The units do not demand anything out of the ordinary, as jogging and some strength training should be in the repertoire of anyone planning to apply to a special unit. Now it is just a case of building up your skills and training specifically for the big day.

These are the requirements of the various units in the German-speaking world:

KOMMANDO SPEZIALKRÄFTE DER MARINE [KSM]

Naval Special Forces Command—Kampfschwimmer Company

- 5,000-meter run in under of 22 minutes
- 1,000-meter swim in under of 24 minutes
- at least 60 seconds of apnea diving
- at least 30 meters of distance diving (with a turn)
- at least 8 pull-ups with an overhand grip (pronation)
- 15 × 100-pounds bench press
- Basic Fitness Test (BFT)

In a second phase, physical fitness is tested by means of a very demanding, multi-day endurance exercise, known as “Hell Week” for obvious reasons.

KOMMANDO SPEZIALKRÄFTE [KSK]

German Special Forces Command

- 5 pull-ups with an overhand grip and dead hangs
- physical fitness test
- doing the obstacle course in field uniform and helmet in under 1:40 minutes
- 7-kilometer cross-country run in field uniform with 20 kg of load in under 52 minutes
- swimming 500 meters in under 15 minutes

SPEZIALEINSATZKOMMANDO [SEK]

Special Task Forces of the German Police

- 3,000-meter run in under 13 minutes
- bench press, pull-ups, and dips with dead hangs (at least 10 repetitions)
- boxing (to test self-defense abilities and willpower)
- obstacle course (constantly changing obstacles)
- height test
- team task
- swimming test, clothed, combination exercise in the water (e.g., diving, rescue, climbing out of the water on a rope, dismantling and assembling a weapon underwater, staying afloat without using your hands, etc.)

Please note that the requirements may vary depending on the federal state.

GRENZSCHUTZGRUPPE 9 DER BUNDESPOLIZEI (GSG 9)

Border Guard Group 9 of the Federal Police

- Cooper test
- 100-meter run in under 13.4 seconds
- standing jump of at least 2.40 m
- at least 10 pull-ups with an overhand grip and dead hangs
- bench-pressing 75 percent of one's own body weight, at least 10 repetitions
- indoor course with 14 obstacles
- endurance run with a concentration test

JAGDKOMMANDO

Commandos of the Austrian Armed Forces

- 8-kilometer footslog with a 20 kg backpack over undulating terrain in under 60 minutes
- 30-meter rope climb
- 300-meter swim (fully dressed, without shoes) in under 11 minutes
- 10-meter jump into water upon command without hesitation
- obstacle course in under 5.10 minutes
- performance and willingness to perform in the context of an endurance exercise
- combat skills
- psychological, sensorimotor aptitude test
- passing a full-contact fight
- A-E test: 6 pull-ups in 60 seconds, 48 squats in 120 seconds, 31 press-ups in 120 seconds, 25 sit-ups in 120 seconds, 19 squat jumps in 60 seconds, 2,400-meter run in under 12 minutes

KOMMANDO SPEZIALKRÄFTE DER SCHWEIZER ARMEE [KSK CH]

Swiss Special Forces Command – here: AAD10

- 50 push-ups without interruption
- 60 trunk bends without interruption
- 10 pull-ups with an overhand grip without interruption
- 5 km cross-country run in sportswear in under 24 minutes
- 8 km footslog in a camouflage suit and field boots with 15 kg of load in under 58 minutes
- 25 km fast march in a camouflage suit and field boots with 25 kg of load in under 3.5 hours
- 300-meter swim in under 10 minutes

NEVER BACK

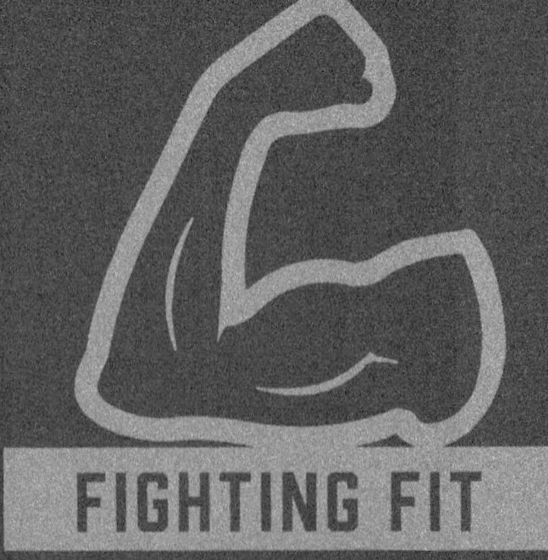

FURTHER READING

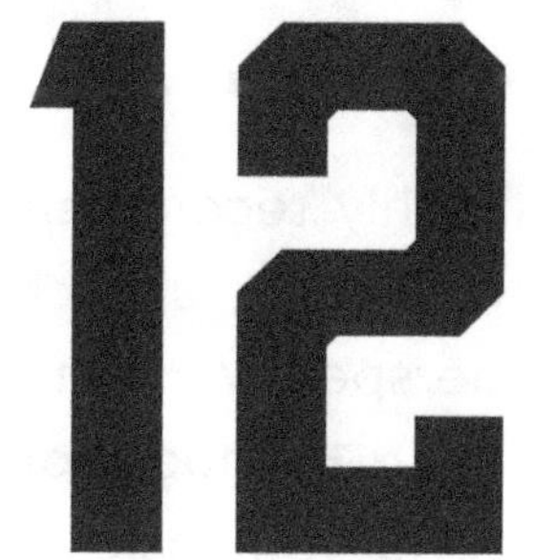

BOOKS AND WEBSITES ON THE SUBJECT OF FITNESS ARE A DIME A DOZEN.

Many of these books also pull the wool over your eyes. Here we present a small selection of books that we think could either be interesting for you or are rather pointless.

+ FIT ON DUTY: FITNESS IN THE POLICE SERVICE (in German)

The complete package from the perspective of Ralf Schmidt. He is a police officer from specialized sections of the CID as well as an athlete, trainer, and instructor. You will find various chapters that are also very interesting for soldiers. E.g., sports after (duty) injuries, over-40 service sport and sports, in action under difficult conditions. Above all, however, ranks the preparation for the selection procedures of various special forces.

Highly recommended as an addition to your book collection, as Schmidt describes training from the perspective of necessity. Keeping it real is the key word. He does not try to sell you anything but instead gives you basic ideas that you should consider as an officer or soldier in order to be operational. This also includes preparation for special forces training.

RALF SCHMIDT, FIT ON DUTY. FITNESS IM POLIZEIDIENST
S. Ka. Verlag, Nuremberg, 2018, 225 page (in German)

+ THE BUNDESWEHR COMBAT SWIMMER

Christin-Désirée Rudolph followed the combat swimmers for a long time. In addition to informative facts about the operation teams, she also describes the training very extensively and documents it with lots of text and pictures. This gives you a very good impression of the various tasks that await you during training. Take a look at the photos. The expressions on the trainees' faces speak volumes. If you cannot imagine pushing yourself to the limit in the same way, then it is better not to apply. A great book to add to your collection.

CHRISTIN-DÉSIRÉE RUDOLPH, DIE KAMPFSCHWIMMER DER BUNDESWEHR
Motorbuch Verlag, Stuttgart, 2014, 176 pages (in German)

+ PERSEVERANCE: MENTAL AND PHYSICAL TRAINING OF ELITE UNITS

This book by Alexander Stilwell shows how elite soldiers develop their extraordinary stamina. With simple step-by-step instructions for physical exercises, mental techniques, survival, and close combat techniques. It is not particularly suitable when preparing for a selection process, which is not what it was written for. It might, however, be a good idea to get a different perspective on perseverance, because that is what ultimately matters during training.

ALEXANDER STILWELL, THE SAS AND ELITE FORCES MANUAL OF MENTAL & PHYSICAL ENDURANCE: HOW TO REACH YOUR PHYSICAL AND MENTAL PEAK
Griffin, 2006, 192 pages

+ THE PATH OF DISCIPLINE

Controlling your thoughts, self-discipline, and strength are the keywords in this book by Jocko Willink, a retired Navy SEAL officer. The full title is *Discipline Equals Freedom: Field Manual: Mk1 MOD1.* Willink does not provide any techniques, and the book is not a guidebook in the classic sense, but it offers almost meditative texts that are intended to guide people to accept and learn discipline as a path to freedom. In other words, there are no shortcuts on this path. Your performance is decisive. A great book that you can pick up again and again to read a page and reflect. Jocko Willink also has a great podcast that is always about one thing, namely leadership and discipline: *jockopodcast.com*

JOCKO WILLINK, DISCIPLINE EQUALS FREEDOM: FIELD MANUAL: MK1 MOD1
St. Martin's Press, 2020, 256 pages

+ BE STRONG

"Strong people are harder to kill, and more useful in general." (Mark Rippetoe) Here we go again! The massed ranks of fitness books and guides have now been joined by another one—or rather, it has been around for a while. But this is not like the other books. Neither in style nor in approach, nor in price.

This book is about getting stronger. And it does so comprehensively. It should be clear to everyone by now that strength training in one form or another is essential for soldiers. Fitness is good and important in everyday combat, but it is of little use if you have to rescue your comrade, carry heavy equipment, or survive close combat situations. We need strength for this; the more, the better. And this book shows us how to get it. It was written by a wrestler, which is a nice touch because wrestling is the basis of modern military hand-to-hand combat. An active wrestler also has the opportunity to constantly measure his strength against others and can therefore enjoy following their development both in absolute and relative terms. Another point in which this book differs from many others is that, as the title suggests, it endeavors to build strength and is therefore not explicitly designed for bodybuilding.

As wrestlers naturally have to be careful not to drop out of their weight class, but at the same time be as strong and agile as possible, this book has many useful tips to get the most out of your body without unnecessarily bulking up. It is also to the book's credit that you can read it and work with it even as an absolute beginner, even if a certain basic level of experience in the gym is certainly not a disadvantage concerning a better understanding of some things. The writing style is informal and relaxed, which makes it extremely entertaining and motivates the reader. The most important topics, such as basic exercises, training with simple means (Bulgarian bag), body weight exercises, kettlebells, nutrition, interval training, and many more, are presented to the reader in a thoroughly enjoyable way. Finally, there is a large amount of further reading in the appendix. Our conclusion: one of the best books available today.

JOHN FLAIS, SEI STARK!
is available as a free download (also for Kindle or as a PDF). Print it out, make notes, and take it with you to training. Download here: https://archive.org/details/Flais-SeiStark1_1 (in German)

+ FIT WITHOUT EQUIPMENT: EXERCISING WITH YOUR BODY WEIGHT

Regarding content, Mark Lauren's books are very good. Unfortunately, he also promises that you can prepare yourself for the selection process and service in elite units with four training sessions and exercises using only your own body weight (calisthenics). Anyone who has read this paperback carefully will realize that not everyone can prepare in this way. Again, take what you need, because the exercises he presents are excellent and can enhance and even enrich your own training.

MARK LAUREN AND JOSHUA CLARK, YOU ARE YOUR OWN GYM: THE BIBLE OF BODYWEIGHT EXERCISES
Orleans Publishing, 192 pages

Mark Lauren also has a website with additional information on his training concept:
marklauren.com

+ FIT WITHOUT EQUIPMENT: FUEL

Eat like the cavemen did. Paleo diet is the trend Mark Lauren illustrates here. And it works. I have never tried it myself, but I know a few soldiers who have been trying it for years and are now "living" it. The concept involves a complete change of diet and is not a quick fix. But it is also an extreme restriction in this day and age. The range of products on offer in supermarkets is huge and not always healthy. Above all, you need to understand how carbohydrates, proteins, and fats work and interact with each other. This requires that you familiarize yourself with the subject thoroughly.

What I do not agree with is his statement that your entire fitness level, appearance, strength, etc. will improve simply because of this diet. Unfortunately, he fails to mention that all of his students also do a lot of sports. You should be aware of this if you decide to buy his book.

With this book, you realize that there is a lot of work at the beginning and that you have to completely change your usual eating routine. If you want to do this, this is the ideal method for you.

MARK LAUREN, BODY FUEL: CALORIE-CYCLE YOUR WAY TO REDUCED BODY FAT AND GREATER MUSCLE DEFINITION
Ballantine Books, 340 pages

+ THE U.S. NAVY SEAL GUIDE TO FITNESS AND NUTRITION

This book, with its almost 500 pages, is a Navy SEAL nutrition guide. A few of the 10 nutrition tips appealed to me because they are very simple and easy to implement.

They are the basics for people who have not yet dealt with the subject of nutrition in depth. However, most of these 10 tips form the basis for a good start in the world of nutrition:

1. Do not believe anything written about nutrition by someone trying to sell you something.
2. Read the labels on food packaging. Carbohydrates, proteins, and the amount of fat per serving are listed there.
3. Most people do not need to take extra vitamins. But if you want to increase your vitamin intake, take inexpensive products that can be consumed daily. The megadoses of expensive "miracle" vitamins only increase the vitamin content of what you excrete every day.
4. Do not supplement with proteins or amino acids. Two grams of protein per kilogram of body weight is the highest recommended amount of protein (even for weightlifting and bodybuilding). Most athletes who are not vegetarians consume more than this in their normal diet.

5. Reduce the fat content of your diet to 30 percent (1 gram of fat = 9 calories). Red meat, peanuts, hard cheese, and anything deep-fried. This is what you need to watch out for.
6. If endurance is required, e.g., during long operations, cold diving days or triathlons, top up your carbohydrate reserves three days, before the event, starting with 1,500 calories per day. Reduce your fat and protein intake at the same time. Also, reduce your training on these days and avoid exposing yourself to the cold.
7. For long, intensive aerobic training sessions (Basic Underwater Demolition/SEAL or triathlon), eat enough carbohydrates to maintain your weight. The best sources are pasta, fruit, bread, potatoes, and rice.
8. Eat fresh fruit, fresh vegetables, and whole-meal products every day.
9. Short-term weight loss diets are generally pointless and sometimes dangerous. A lasting change in your weight can only be achieved through a sustainable change in your diet and exercise behavior.
10. The most common nutritional problem is overeating. Do not eat when you are not hungry. Stop eating when you are full, not when the plate is empty.

THE U.S. NAVY SEAL GUIDE TO FITNESS AND NUTRITION
Skyhorse Publishing, 2007, 496 pages

+ BECOMING A SUPPLE LEOPARD

Kelly Starret's book is already available in an expanded edition. This makes the book easier to understand, with more clearly explained movement patterns, a clearer golden thread, explanatory sketches, and explained foreign words.

This book must be read and understood in its entirety in order to be able to fully implement Starret's training concept. However, it is also possible to extract individual chapters, e.g., the mobilization section. Unfortunately, this book cannot be described in a few sentences. It is simply too complex. It covers tension patterns, muscle alignment, and the mobilization already mentioned. But above all, injury prevention and pain relief are at the top of the list. A few supplementary YouTube videos offer quite good summaries.

From the point of view of preparing for SOF, there is a lot to be gained here, but not for everyone. It is also a very time-consuming process. It is intended more as a guideline for a sensible, healthy, and correct approach to all kinds of sports exercises. Personally, this book does not really help me. Over the years, I have acquired my own understanding of training and regeneration and managed it so well that I do not want to adopt any other concept.

KALLY STARRETT AND GLEN CORDOZA, BECOMING A SUPPLE LEOPARD: THE ULTIMATE GUIDE TO RESOLVING PAIN, PREVENTING INJURY, AND OPTIMIZING ATHLETIC PERFORMANCE
Victory Belt Publishing, pages

+ MILITARY FITNESS: TRAIN LIKE A KAMPFSCHWIMMER

Military Fitness: Train Like a Kampfschwimmer written by Andreas Aumann and myself, describes a type of fitness training that has been around for centuries. Even the commanders of old were aware that soldiers during campaigns or a siege (which often lasted months) had to remain fit. One therefore relied on simple aids and body weight, as soldiers could not be expected to bring along their own training equipment. It is exactly this problem we are still faced with today: For soldiers on training courses, managers and fitters away on business, people who do not like gyms, or sportspeople who have discovered calisthenics this book can be a first step towards successful low-hassle workouts anywhere. To this end, we have limited ourselves to workouts with slings, kettlebells, and sandbags, as well as exercises involving partners or body weight.

Can this book be used to prepare yourself for an SOF? Only to a limited degree. As I have often stated concerning the other books, there are some helpful hints here. As the book not only consists of exercises, the part dealing with training theory is very interesting. The exercises, however, are not intended to prepare for SOF selection procedures. Our book deals with military fitness in the original sense, as described above. I can, however, recommend it to anybody who wants to lay the groundwork in this field. We have included 370 pictures of the exercises and training plans, and have written a very informative chapter on military fitness. The part on training theory, which is very important to me, is written in a clear style, and every exercise can be extended and scaled up.

TORSTEN SCHREIBER AND ANDREAS AUMANN, MILITARY FITNESS: TRAINIEREN WIE DIE KAMPFSCHWIMMER
Meyer und Meyer Verlag, Munich, 2015, 290 pages
(in German)

+ MENTAL POWER FOR EXTREME SITUATIONS

I highly recommend this book, because mental power is an important factor in succeeding in an elite unit. Clemens Clausen, a former combat swimmer, security, adviser, and trainer in maritime security knows what he is talking about. He faced many extreme situations and, with this book, has found a good way to show the way towards improvement and mastery. Fortunately, it also shows that it is sometimes not possible to be mentally strong enough to master every situation. And that mental power cannot be acquired in a few days or weeks. It takes a while. Which is an important point this book makes.

CLEMENS CLAUSEN, MENTALKRAFT: MENTALE STÄRKE FÜR EXTREMSITUATIONEN
Books on Demand, 2022

CONCLUSION

If you are into these kinds of books, buy them. Do not, however, believe everything they tell you, because some types of training or mental exercises are not suitable for everybody. Use what you need for your training. I personally recommend *Fit on duty. Fitness im Polizeidienst* and *Die Kampfschwimmer der Bundeswehr.*

I am not a fan of learning ever more new and fashionable types of training. Discussions regarding the pros and cons of traditional techniques grate on my nerves because scientific statistics are disproved every five years. I have read some books because I need to be flexible as a trainer and expand my horizons. I have, however, found that, barring individual exercises, there is almost nothing new I can learn from them. My traditional type of training works perfectly. On the contrary, the many sweeping statements, which often do not even apply to many sportspeople, must be seen as a sales pitches that, in the final analysis, disappoint. Especially if you remember that many authors have excellent licenses, degrees, and lots of experience.

Much more effective, therefore, is a trainer who adapts to your individual, physical performance, integrates this into customized training plans, and produces analyses by identifying, discussing, and remedying mistakes, as well as adapting the training plan to your current status every couple of months.

DO IT, AND DON'T JUST READ. ONLY THEN WILL YOU SUCCEED.

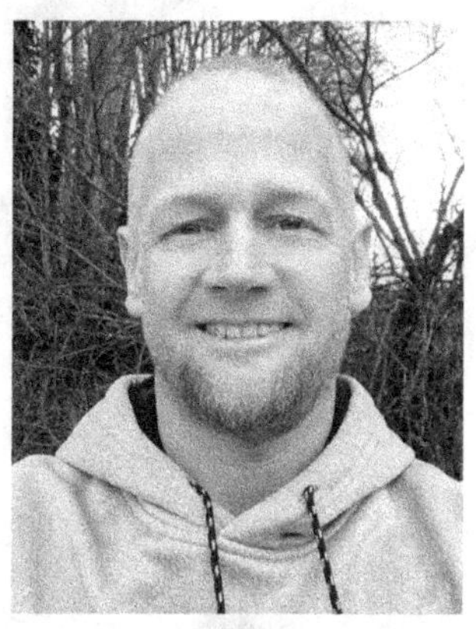

TORSTEN SCHREIBER [BORN 1979]

is a "Kampfschwimmer" – a German Navy SEAL – and boasts over twenty years of experience as a triathlete. During his active service, he had to train intensively. On the topic of military sports, he co-authored the book *Military Fitness: Training Like A Kampfschwimmer* (with Andreas Aumann). As a PT instructor, he prepares athletes for a wide range of performance goals.

For several years, he has volunteered in the field of personnel recruitment via social media. In this book, he shares his knowledge of efficient preparation with individuals who want to meet the SOF challenge.

The author:
www.instagram.com/todde_439

Association of German Combat Swimmers:
www.instagram.com/kampfschwimmer_eckernfoerde

Printed in the USA
CPSIA information can be obtained
at www.ICGtesting.com
CBHW052358031024
15325CB00034B/192

9 783903 526082